SWNHS

C20105031

3 WM
30
SHE

Rw
6113

Mental Health Work
in the Community:
Theory and Practice in
Social Work and
Community Psychiatric
Nursing

UNIVERSITY OF PLYMOUTH
LIBRARY SERVICES

FHSW

D0317710

Mental Health Work in the Community: Theory and Practice in Social Work and Community Psychiatric Nursing

Michael Sheppard

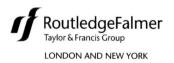

RoutledgeFalmer
Taylor & Francis Group

LONDON AND NEW YORK

© Michael Sheppard 1991

All rights reserved. No part of this publication may be reproduced, stored in a retrieval system, or transmitted, in any form or by any means, electronic, mechanical, photocopyright, recording, or otherwise, without permission in writing from the Publisher.

First Published 1991
By Routledge Falmer, 11 New Fetter Lane, London, EC4P 4EE.

Transferred to Digital Printing 2004

British Library Cataloging in Publication Data
Sheppard, Michael
   Mental health work in the community.
   1. Mentally disordered persons. Community care
   I. Title
   616.8903

   ISBN 1–85000–978–3
   1–85000–979–1 pbk

Library of Congress Cataloging-in-Publication Data

Printed and bound by Antony Rowe Ltd, Eastbourne

Contents

Preface

This book presents a comparative analysis of the work of mental health social workers and community psychiatric nurses. Both professions lay claim, to a considerable degree, to the same 'territory', and, in view of developments in community care, the examination of the relative merits of the claims of these professions to this territory, is of considerable importance. The findings, which are ultimately favourable to social workers, are bound to be controversial, since occupations do not generally willingly leave territory to which they have previously laid claim. This, however, cannot be helped, and I have attempted to be scrupulously fair by working with meanings common to both professions.

Had I realized the size of the task I had set myself at the outset, I might have hesitated to embark on this project. It involved not only the comparison of two professions, but also both the detailed examination of the theoretical foundations of both professions and the empirically researched examination of practice. However, the findings potentially have far reaching implications for policy and practice in the mental health field, and they address issues which are likely to remain significant for the foreseeable future. Additionally, however, this book presents a further contribution to a debate in which I have previously been involved: the relationship between theory and practice (and particularly the place of the social sciences) in social work.

I have been helped by a number of people in preparation of this book. My colleagues George Giarchi and Pamela Abbott have discussed various aspects with me. Terry Mangles has been free with his time in giving me both statistical and computing advice. Ted White of Manchester University's Department of Nursing helpfully discussed various aspects of community psychiatric nursing. Chapman-Hall were kind enough to send me an advanced copy of Charles Brooker's *Community Psychiatric Nursing: A Research Perspective*. I am most grateful of all to Sheryl Lester and her social work team, and Chris Bulley and his CPN team for their involvement in this project. They inevitably gave an enormous amount of time to this project, and it goes without saying that without them it simply would not have happened. Finally, I wish to thank my typists, and in particular, Sally Petherick and Sue Ellicott who typed the bulk of the book. I alone, of course, am responsible for any errors which may appear.

Chapter 1

Introduction

The context for the practice of social work and community psychiatric nursing (CPN) as well as the development of community mental health centres (CMHC) is provided by the increasing emphasis since 1945 on community care of the mentally ill. To a large degree this arose from the development of psychotropic drugs in the 1950s, which revolutionized the control of major mental illness, such as schizophrenia, creating an atmosphere of therapeutic optimism. This was allied to a growing disenchantment with hospitals as an appropriate setting for managing mental illness, and the potential debilitating effect of institutional care (Goffman, 1961). The term 'institutional neurosis' described a process by which hospital regimes created individuals with characteristics such as submissiveness, apathy and a shuffling gait (Barton, 1959). Closely associated with this was the preferred notion of 'normalization': 'The conviction that if people with handicaps are treated like everyone else, their handicaps will cease to be of importance to them and to society' (Jones, 1988, p. 90). In political terms the focus for decarceration of patients was most evident in Powell's well known speech as Minister of Health planning to halve the number of hospital beds in fifteen years (Powell, 1961), which was followed by the 'Hospital Plan', which envisaged the run down and eventual closure of existing hospitals and their replacement by short stay psychiatric units and community care facilities provided by local authorities (Ministry of Health, 1962). Figures for bed occupancy reflect the subsequent reduced emphasis on institutional care: average daily bed occupancy reduced from 118,800 in 1966 to 83,800 in 1976 and 61,500 in 1986 (Department of Health, 1988).

While reduced hospital care focused primarily on major mental illness, research has identified high levels of morbidity, primarily in minor mental illness, in general population surveys. The point prevalence of psychiatric disorder is somewhere between 90 and 200 per 1000 at risk, primarily constituting various combinations of depression and anxiety (Goldberg and Huxley, 1980). These disorders arise in a social context and rates, notably of depression, are about twice as high for women as men, and higher in urban than traditional rural contexts. (Brown and Harris, 1978; Brown *et al.*, 1977). While Goldberg and Huxley (1980) assert community depression is generally less severe than that encountered in hospital, research by Brown and his colleagues (1985) indicates that, except for a small proportion of severely depressed, depression in the community is as severe as that in hospital. The implications of research were not simply the discovery of high levels of morbidity, but that much of it goes untreated.

The growing emphasis on care in the community was accompanied by the establishment of Social Services Departments in 1971, followed by National Health Service reorganization in 1974 with the associated organizational separation of social work from health professionals. Workers formerly concentrating on mental health, child care, elderly and handicapped work respectively, were brought together in one unified social work profession. The effect was to create two empires, one social work based in local authorities and the other, dominated by medicine, based in health authorities, Together with the other developments in community care, this generated a number of issues evident in subsequent policy documents. The first was interprofessional collaboration, recognized increasingly as a problem with organizational separation. The 1975 White Paper (DHSS, 1975a) advocated the attachment of social workers to primary care teams as well as their involvement in specialist multiprofessional psychiatric teams, the advantages of which were closer collaboration and the pooling of a variety of perspectives and skills. A later document (DHSS, 1978) charted the problematic nature of collaboration deriving from differences in organization, knowledge and status, and suggested joint work, bringing together different skills in the service of particular clients, as superior to individual work.

A further issue relates to medical and non-medical approaches, which the White Paper (DHSS, 1975a) considered partly competing and partly complementary. Hence, the belief in the importance of biochemical factors and the efficacy of drug treatment was contrasted with approaches stressing underlying social, psychological and environmental causes of mental illness, particularly neurotic problems. The alternative to competing positions was an eclectic approach incorporating biological, psychological and social elements. The competing positions tend to emphasize to different degrees 'medical' and 'non-medical' approaches. A third, associated, issue relates to prevention. Primary prevention was considered in broad terms of reducing individuals' exposure to social circumstances likely to place their mental health at risk. Concern was expressed about early recognition, assessment and support for those caring for the mentally ill, involving not just professionals but employers, managers and planners (DHSS, 1975a). A fourth issue related to the target group. The Social Services Committee (Short, 1985) contrasted the concern with decarcerated patients with the non-hospitalized mentally ill in the community. They commented on the 'almost obsessive concentration' in public policy on the former group, and suggested the balance should be redressed by a greater involvement with the latter. To a considerable degree this entailed a change in the balance of emphasis: from major mental illness, predominantly associated with hospitalization, to minor mental illness, predominating in the community. Throughout, there has been a concern that political and financial commitment to community care has been more rhetorical than practical, and concerns have been expressed that community care should not be viewed as a cheap option (Short, 1985; Audit Commission, 1986). These concerns have not been dispelled with the publication of the White Paper (Department of Health, 1989) giving primary responsibility, as suggested in previous reports, to local authorities (Jones, 1988).

Community Mental Health Centres (CMHCs)

CMHCs represent an important response to the development of care in the community. Echlin (1988, p. 2) comments that

> Judging from the evidence of the rapid expansion of CMHCs in Britain in recent years, planners are increasingly turning to CMHCs as their favoured method for moving mental health provision out of hospital.

The first centre was opened in 1977, since when there has been an exponential growth: by 1987, 122 centres existed or had planned funding, and 155 were at the unfunded planning stage (Craig *et al.*, 1990). Most authorities possessed, or planned, CMHCs (Sayce, 1987). The inspiration came largely from American (and Italian) experience, where CMHCs arose within the Civil Rights movement of the 1960s, but subsequently suffered both political and service delivery problems (Jones, 1988). However, unlike their American counterparts, British CMHCs have no mandated services: their development stemmed rather from enthusiasm and commitment. There is, however, no simple definition of a CMHC. Sayce (1989) comments that the CMHC has become something of a buzzword, reflecting the belief that, even if an authority did not have one, they nonetheless *should*. But a cursory glance at British developments shows a bewildering variety: mental health advice centres, mental health resource centres, day centres, community mental health teams as well as those avoiding explicit reference to mental health in their title (hoping to reduce stigma) (Sayce, 1988).

Echlin (1988) identifies two models. The first is a base or building in the community for a multidisciplinary team serving a prescribed catchment area. Others see a central base as a barrier to service provision and work instead peripatetically in different settings such as community centres, church halls and health centres. Dick (1985) also identifies two models as approaches to managing psychiatric morbidity. The first is a service acting as a 'funnel', passing most work to local resources (e.g. primary health care, social services) and only maintains that which cannot otherwise be managed. The second is a specialist service providing particular styles of treatment: however if the particular skills available do not match client needs, the client cannot be helped. It is service driven rather than client need led. Sayce (1987) identifies three approaches: first, as an entry point for most of the locality's mental health referrals to a devolved psychiatric service; second, a sessional model offering counselling and/or group work; third, a community development model, with an emphasis on initiating formal and informal networks of care.

Although models may differ, there are common characteristics for which CMHCs strive. *Accessibility* is the first (Peck and Joyce, 1985). This contains a number of elements: potential clients should have direct access to the service rather than requiring intermediate referral by professionals ('walk-in service'); the service response should be as speedy as possible; the premises should be geographically easily available, either being local or on major transport routes; and stigma should be reduced (encouraging referral) by using non-stigmatizing (ordinary) buildings and service titles. Second, CMHCs tend to emphasize *psychosocial* rather than medical (biophysical) methods of intervention. This involves an emphasis on social and familial dimensions, and a greater available range of therapies and intervention provided in a coordinated way which would be unavailable (without attachments) in GP services. Third, *multidisciplinary teamwork* is emphasized. For some, this involves greater equality, rather than medical leadership, between involved professions. It certainly emphasizes greater cooperation and collaboration between mental health workers. Most centres are based around CPNs and social workers, and some advocate the development of generic mental health professionals, because of apparently overlapping skills and consequent 'role blurring' (Peck and Joyce, 1985; Jones, 1988) which, it is argued, makes demarcation by professional group obsolete. Fourth, *comprehensiveness* is often emphasized. In part this relates to multidisciplinary teams offering various skills, and it may be more accurate to describe CMHCs as part of a comprehensive service (Sayce, 1989). Finally *community links* are often considered important. This can involve links with other agencies, such as 'outposting' to general practice (Grey *et al.*, 1988). It can also involve taking seriously consumers' views of the service, through, for example, consumer studies, or even consumer participation in the planning and development of CMHCs.

Social Work and Community Psychiatric Nursing

Although social work has a history going back to the nineteenth century, it dates back in its modern form to 1971. Prior to this, with the establishment of Social Services Departments, social work was fragmented into separate groups, and Mental Welfare Officers (MWOs) were local authority based, while Psychiatric Social Workers (PSWs) were hospital based. MWOs were incorporated into the new departments in 1971, followed in 1974 by PSWs, with NHS reorganization. Removal from medical oversight and incorporating PSWs into the professional mainstream might be considered beneficial. However, other 'immediate consequences were well nigh catastrophic' (Hargreaves, 1979, p. 77). Although Seebohm did not condemn specialization, the word 'generic' (referring to skills or knowledge common to different aspects of work) was misused, and redefined as 'generalist' with the 'unrealistic expectation that all social workers should be professionally competent in dealing with every kind of human problem and need' (Sainsbury, 1977, p. 77). This had various effects on mental health work. To a considerable extent this meant the loss of previously available specialist mental health skills. Hargreaves (1979, p. 77) calculated there was a reduction of a third in social work person-hours devoted specifically to mental health between 1967 and 1976. He set this against an increase of 35 per cent in the number of psychiatric nurses during the same period. Together with the loss of specialist skills, the interprofessional relationship between doctors and social workers generally worsened. Psychiatrists and PSWs/MWOs had formerly had close professional relationships based on a high degree of specialization and common concerns, which were disrupted by reorganization. This loss was frequently accompanied by drifting apart and disillusionment. Third, mental health was given a relatively low priority by the new departments, which were increasingly dominated — particularly with child abuse deaths — by child care. The recent White Paper (Department of Health, 1989) comments on the still small fraction of SSD budgets devoted to mental health.

Although this era was dominated by a generalist orientation, many ex-MWOs maintained an interest in mental health work and were able to continue with this as an aspect of their caseload (Howe, 1986). More recently widespread reorganization by individual SSDs has led to increases in specialist interests, with a realization that expertise in all aspects of social work is unrealistic. Reorganization has occurred either at a department wide level, with changes associated with central policy, or on a 'bottom up' basis where changes, occurring at area team level, are decided by the area teams themselves. This has taken three forms: structural changes in teams involving specialist subgroups, a growth in the number of individual specialist mental health posts, and bias in individual workers' caseloads, whereby 75 per cent of cases involve a particular client group (Challis and Fairlie, 1986, 1987). From a position of virtual abandonment of mental health posts following the 1971 reorganization, there has been a drift back to more specialist work in more recent years, and the growth of specialism has been marked in mental health. This process is likely to be emphasized with the effects of changes presaged in the 1989 White Paper.

Community psychiatric nursing is a relatively recent development. According to Hunter (1974) the first recorded service began at Warlingham Park Hospital, Croydon, and services began at Moorhaven, Devon in 1985. The impetus for a community service arose, according to Hunter, from informal contacts with patients' relatives and the influx of ex-service person-nel with extensive life experiences outside the mental hospital. They were subject to haphazard development, and by 1966, forty-two hospitals used nursing staff in community work. The remarkable growth of CPN services followed local government reorganization and the emphasis on generalist social work. This appears not to be coincidental. The Community Psychiat-ric Nursing Association (CPNA) representatives giving evidence to the Social Services Committee (Short, 1985) commented that, with the loss of specialist expertise and the resulting gaps in social work provision, CPNs moved into a vacuum created by 'the genericism (sic) of social work'. This may not have been the only factor: it is noticeable that the growth in the number of CPNs occurred contemporaneous with the decline in the number of hospital beds, reflecting an increased emphasis on community care.

It is difficult to identify the exact growth in CPN numbers, although while they were hardly mentioned in the 1975 White Paper *Better Services for the Mentally Ill* (DHSS, 1975a) they were considered important in the 1985 Short Report, reflecting their much higher profile. By 1980 there were 1667 CPNs employed nationally, a figure which rose to 2758 (a 66 per cent increase) by 1985 (CPNA, 1985b). However, while the 1985 ratio of CPN:population was 1:23,800, the CPNA aim was for 1:10,000, indicating further developments, 'warmly welcomed' by the Short Report (1985). However, the overall figure concealed considerable variations in CPN pro-vision between different regions. Parnell (1978) noted considerable variation also in the organization of services, reflected in the 1985 National Survey. Thus while the majority of CPNs worked in general psychiatry teams, 29 per cent worked in a specialist capacity, the majority with the elderly. Further-more, their organizational base varied: the largest group (though declining relative to others) were based in psychiatric hospitals (37 per cent) while others, each comprising between 16 and 19 per cent of CPNs, were based in DGH psychiatric units, health centres and 'other' bases (CPNA, 1985b).

Role

Social work, as the better established occupation has a role, the core of which is well established, although it has developed over time. Although recognized as largely determined by the profession, their role has nonetheless been outlined in official documents. The Ottan Report (DHSS, 1975b) identified various elements to health social workers' role: the assessment of social factors contributing to diagnosis; providing advice on social factors and approaches contributing to treatment; assessing social factors affecting dis-charge from hospital; and provision of, if necessary, long term after care support. Additionally in the primary health setting the role advocated in-cluded therapeutic work with individuals, families or groups; mobilizing practical resources and liaison with outside agencies; educating the team on social factors in health care; and specialist consultant to social services staff. The White Paper (DHSS, 1975a) discussed the social work role specifically in relation to mental health, identifying three main areas. First, they should have a working knowledge of symptoms, treatment, cause and prognosis of an individual's illness. Second, therapeutic work with individuals and families involves developing and maintaining a consistent relationship with the individual, knowing the ways the family may be affected, being aware of their particular family relationships and offering psychological and practical support to them. Third, they identify the use and mobilization of support services and outside agencies, such as primary health care, social security, housing, social services, and the ability to judge not just what is viable but also apply professional skill in considering what is best for each client.

Subsequent developments have expanded upon this traditional social work role. The Barclay Report (National Institute for Social Work [NISW], 1982), a semi-official document, advocated the development of community social work. Beyond concerns with individuals and families, this advocated the use and development of social networks, involving a partnership between social services, informal carers and voluntary agencies. Its focus is upon actual or potential links which exist or could be fostered between those with similar concerns. Two broad categories are identified: the first involves a focus on locality in which particular interests are related to geographical area, while the second is distinguished by a shared concern or problem, e.g. the needs of particular client groups. The report identified the need for social workers to increase their capacity to negotiate and bargain, to act as individual and group advocates, and recognize and use communities of interest between different people. This of course involved roles general to social work rather than specific to mental health. More recently the 1989 White Paper has outlined a further role, that of case manager, likely to be taken on primarily, but not entirely, by social workers. Where complex needs exist (e.g. chronic mental health problems) case managers may ensure that individuals' needs are regularly reviewed, act as assessor of care needs, plan and secure delivery of care, monitor the care provided and review client needs. Case management will be linked to budgetary responsibility and occur in the context of a range of resources. Finally, social work contains the specialist role of Approved Social Worker, primarily involving assessment for compulsory admission, unique to the profession, which has been discussed in detail elsewhere (Sheppard, 1990).

To a considerable degree, the role ascribed to themselves by CPNs overlaps with that of social workers. There are, however, no descriptions of the CPN's role in official documents (which social workers have), and there is some lack of professional clarity. The Short Report (1985) stated that 'it is in need of self discipline and definition' commenting that not just health managers, but many CPNs are uncertain about their role (vol 1, para 193). Early statements of the CPN role were relatively limited, reflecting a 'medical handmaid' service: the provision of basic nursing care (medically supervised), supervision of prescribed medication, consultant to non-psychiatric nurses, keeping close contact with PSWs and other agencies, and providing reassurance and encouragement to individuals and their families, although significantly problems involving family dynamics were to be immediately referred to the PSW (Greene, 1968; Moore, 1964). Such modest representations of the practical nurse did not long survive social work reorganization. Hunter (1974) identified additional to continuing care, the provision of psychotherapeutic treatment, crisis intervention, groupwork and behaviour therapy with increasing emphasis on group and interpersonal dynamics.

Recent conceptions of CPNs' role demonstrates further its similarity with mental health social work. The CPNA recognized CPNs required 'techniques and strategies' previously associated with other professions, and even used the social work term 'good casework' to identify desired practice (CPNA, 1985a, p. 7). They are concerned 'with people's emotions' (p. 11), the way they behave, the expression of feelings through individual and groupwork, and helping families explore their problems. In their evidence to the Social Services Committee (Short, 1985) the CPNA drew on two authors; Sladden (1979), who considered CPNs distinguished by their (ubiquitous) ability to operate within the medical, social and psychological frame of reference and Carr *et al.* (1980). The latter provide a description of the CPN role remarkably similar to the traditional social work role, which is divided into six. First, they act as assessor of nursing requirements of patients and families or carers. Second, they offer individual and family psychotherapy. Third, they are managers of their own work, setting priorities and communicating with community agencies. Fourth, they are educators of nurses and other professionals on mental illness. Fifth, they are consultant to nurses and other professionals about nursing care required in specific cases. Finally, they act as clinician — a role not shared with social workers — either basic, monitoring self care and diet, or technical, providing injections and monitoring medication. Thus there is great apparent role overlap: although CPNs may be clinicians, and social workers can be Approved Social Workers.

Role overlap is evident in assessing and working therapeutically with patient and family, working with community agencies and acting in specialist educational and consultant roles. It is most graphically illustrated by those arguing for the common title of community mental health worker. This is advocated by MIND (1983) and has been enthusiastically taken up by some CPNs. Simmons and Brooker (1986), somewhat arrogantly, consider CPNs have been 'sitting on the sidelines waiting for everybody else to catch them up', and consider the title particularly appropriate for CMHCs. However, the British Association of Social Workers (BASW) consider that social work skills are not sufficiently duplicated by CPNs to merit the role blurring inherent from a common title. BASW evidence considered variations in training and knowledge too wide to allow this (Short, 1985, vol III para 1073). The Social Services Committee agreed: 'the general merging and blurring of skills into some kind of "community mental health worker" ... would be unfortunate' (Short, 1985).

Research

Very little published research exists on CMHCs. Most relates to Lewisham Mental Health Advice Centre, constituting a mixture of pamphlets and articles (Bouras and Brough, 1982; Bouras and Tufnall, 1983; Boardman *et al.*, 1987; Boardman and Bouras, 1988). Much of these publications cover the same ground, with updated data. They have two main teams, the Multi-professional Team (MPT), providing an assessment and intervention service, and the Crisis Intervention Team (CIT) available at short notice. The over-whelming majority of both teams' referrals were from health sources, with GPs providing the lion's share but self referrals comprising only 15 per cent of MPT and 3 per cent of CIT referrals. Two thirds of both teams' referrals were for women, but the MPT saw more neurotic and the CIT more psychotic people. The age of MPT clients was more frequently under 40, and more CIT clients were on drugs. Only about two fifths of both groups had a partner, and while nearly half MPT clients received counselling a quarters of CIT clients were hospitalized and a third received mainly domiciliary support or drug therapy. The results showed major differences according to the purpose of the service, with the CIT specializing in particularly disturbed clients. It showed also that it could tap a large pool of untreated, particularly non-psychotic, morbidity. However, low levels of self referrals question its accessibility. Another small retrospective study examined fifty-three self referrals to Eastgate CMHC (Hutton, 1985). The main presenting problems were marital, relationship and anxiety; two fifths dropped out or were referred elsewhere, and others received mainly counselling, group or family therapy. One Coventry study examined client views of a predominantly social work service (Davis *et al.*, 1985). Two thirds felt their goals were mainly or completely achieved and all clients considered counselling very or quite helpful, although only a third felt they were helped with social and economic conditions. Three quarters of clients considered their problems to be somewhat or much better and they cited the relaxed personalized service as particularly welcome.

Mental health social work has been subject to limited research since 1971, and it may broadly be divided into that focusing on Area teams and that focusing on health settings.

Area Teams

A number of studies have examined psychiatric morbidity in social work clients. Huxley and Fitzpatrick (1984) conducted a pilot study using a

9

screening instrument, the general health questionnaire (GHQ), followed by a later more extensive study using the standardized present state examination (PSE), of area team and GP attached social workers. They found 25 per cent of newly referred and consecutively allocated clients were cases, which with threshold cases increased to 53 per cent (Huxley *et al.*, 1987). Corney (1984b) combining the GHQ and standardized clinical interview schedule, studied an intake team and found two thirds to be cases. Cohen and Fisher's (1987) study of a representative sample found, with the widely used 4/5 cut off point, 52 per cent to be cases, and with 10/11, reducing misdiagnosis, 35 per cent. Isaac *et al.* (1986) found 38 per cent of fathers and 56 per cent of mothers who were primary caregivers of children received into care were GHQ cases. Although figures vary, mental health is a major aspect of social work. However, the extent of mental illness has been consistently underestimated. Very few are departmentally designated mental health cases (Corney, 1984b, Huxley *et al.*, 1987), and although social workers identify a mental health problem correctly in half to two thirds of cases (Corney, 1984b: Cohen and Fisher, 1987; Huxley *et al.*, 1987), they show no more than chance ability to diagnose precisely. Overall Huxley *et al.* (1989) conclude that it is important for social workers to understand the nature of psychiatric disability, broadly to recognize and account for it in their work.

Most research of social work intervention suffers from the problem of limited departmental case definition, concentrating only on those defined as mental health cases. Referral shows a fairly consistent pattern: health personnel are major referrers, followed by relatives and friends (Goldburg and Wharburton, 1979; Black *et al.*, 1983). The health origin of referrals may influence client definition as mental health cases. Howe (1986) found emotional and self care, social isolation, familial and financial difficulties to be the most frequently associated problems. Studies show some consistency in work undertaken: investigating and assessing, provision of emotional support and facilitating problem solving are most frequently cited (Howe, 1986; Black *et al.*, 1983). Goldberg and Wharburton (1979) distinguished between short term work — lasting up to one year — and long term work, already on caseloads, and open for at least two years. Of short term cases, 16 per cent were closed after one day and 43 per cent after a month. They were mainly referred at crisis point because a chronic psychiatric illness had upset the family equilibrium. The main work undertaken was assessment and information and advice. With long term work, except in crises, workers largely held a watching brief, and additionally extensively provided assessment, information and advice and emotional sustaining. Outside agencies were frequently contacted, although these were primarily with health agencies and professionals.

One study of social work intervention, not relying on departmental definitions, has been undertaken (Fisher *et al.*, 1984). Clients in three area teams were defined as mentally disordered where impaired mental state or social functioning (a heuristic device) was identified, regardless of agency definition. They combined the examination of referrals with those on longer term caseloads. In relation to the former group, the fairly high proportion of unallocated cases, although often referred to other agencies or appropriately briefly dealt with left, in some cases, a 'cause for concern' because of priorities which prevented their allocation. Of those allocated, 37 per cent were closed within three months and a further 30 per cent within twelve months of referral. Women outnumbered men 2:1 and clients were generally deprived: two fifths were unemployed and those employed were mainly in unskilled or semi-skilled occupations. Of those allocated, only 40 per cent were departmentally defined as mental health cases, the rest being elderly or child and family care. Longer term work was examined through interviews with a sample of clients and workers. They found intervention, averaging over *four years* on open cases, was characterized by unlimited emotionally supportive friendship and practical help rather than being purposive. Clients who felt supported were generally clear about why social workers were visiting, and contact varied according to need. Clients feeling unsupported generally considered social workers had failed to acknowledge fundamental elements of their problems and overlooked areas of personal distress. Social work accounts of work with these clients were divided into monitoring the elderly, supporting socially isolated people and supervising families and children. With the first two groups workers felt they were carrying out a holding operation with little hope of improvement, they considered interviews difficult, and with the socially isolated felt clients lacked motivation for improvement. With families and children workers felt great commitment was necessary, though relationships were profound, and overall they reported greater improvement than with other groups. Overall, however, workers felt much of the work was demoralizing, time consuming and demanding. They also examined relationships with doctors, confirming evidence extensively provided elsewhere, about poor relationships. Workers' approaches to mental health were largely pragmatic, and they showed some suspicion of a 'medical approach', related to a concern about the deleterious effects of labelling. The only circumstances which the majority were prepared to define as mental illness *per se* were those they could not understand, and individuals' behaviour appeared deluded, bizarre and inexplicable.

Health Settings/Specialist Work

Most research on health settings has concentrated on GP attachments. The clientele is, however, different from area teams. Corney's study (1980) showed attachments to have a higher proportion of women, more people aged 16 to 44, and clients living with their families. Referrals were predominantly from health professionals, with a greater proportion of relationships, emotional and mental health problems. Overall attachment scheme clientele were more representative of the general population. Corney (1984b) also examined the mental health of attachment clients using the GHQ and CIS. On both instruments about two thirds of clients were cases, and as in area settings social workers underestimated the extent of mental illness. Cooper *et al.* (1975), and Shepherd *et al.* (1979) undertook a controlled study of attached social work with chronic neurotic clients. They found that, in both clinical and social adjustment scores, social work clients improved significantly more than the control group receiving routine help at one year follow up. Fewer social work clients required psychotropic medication, or were referred for specialist psychiatric help, indicating it was a partial alternative to specialist services. However, the examination of social work activities showed no specific types to be particularly effective. Corney (1984a) studied the effectiveness of attached social workers with depressed women, comparing social work with conventional GP treatment. It comprised two groups: acute — women with symptoms of three months or less — and acute on chronic — (a on c) women with symptoms of more than three months. Overall there were no significant differences between the experimental and control groups in both clinical and social outcome. However, significantly more a on c clients improved in clinical outcome if referred to a social worker, though the reverse was the case for acute clients. There was some evidence that a on c clients improved in social outcome more when referred to a social worker than control group, and they also made fewer demands on their doctor. Clients with poor social contacts and major difficulties with their sexual partners benefited in their clinical though not social scores from social work referral. This was particularly marked in a on c clients. The evidence, then, suggested social work benefits some but hinders other clients. They are most helpful with clients with chronic problems and poor social supports. These clients tended to be more highly motivated, and fared better when given both counselling and practical help.

McAuley *et al.* (1983) reported on the social work task in an acute in-patient unit. This differed from both attachment and area team work. Fewer clients were female or employed than Corney's (1980) attachment clients, although about the same were of working age. Over half had family relations problems, more than Goldberg *et al.*'s (1977) area team group, while like that group over half received some practical help, and information, advice and mobilizing resources were most frequent activities. However, noticeably more in-patient clients received emotional sustaining. Gibbons *et al.* (1978) compared task centred social work (E group) with self poisoning patients with a routine service (C group). Depressive mood fell in both groups, with no significant difference between them, although improvement in social problems was significantly greater in the E group. Repetition of self poisoning showed no significant difference between E and C groups, although client satisfaction at four months was significantly greater in the E group. A further study (Gibbons *et al.*, 1979) examined clients' views in more detail. E clients felt significantly more helped, particularly with their social life, and feeling less upset and disturbed. They were significantly more likely to see their problems as 'better' or 'much better' at follow up (four months). At four months E clients showed significantly more improvement than C clients in social problems, particularly personal and social relations, although differences were not significant at eighteen months. Hudson (1974, 1978) carried out two small studies of behavioural work. With agoraphobic clients (Hudson, 1974) she found clients from well adjusted families had a better prognosis than sick (poorly adjusted) families. Her analysis of work with schizophrenic people involved only five clients, with limited success and only suggestive results (Hudson, 1978).

CPNs have been, if anything, even less subject to case based research than mental health social work. Some studies have attempted to identify the nature of psychiatric disorders on CPN caseloads, although using psychiatrist diagnosis rather than standardized instruments. Sladden's (1979) study of five Edinburgh CPNs found the overwhelming majority (61 per cent) were diagnosed schizophrenic, while depressive and manic depressive clients jointly accounted for 13 per cent. Wooff and her colleagues (Wooff, 1987; Wooff *et al.*, 1986) used case register data to examine the diagnostic make up of CPN clients in Salford. On average between 1976 and 1985 they worked with slightly fewer schizophrenic (28 per cent) than depressed (32 per cent) clients. However, while rates per thousand of both groups grew, the proportion which were schizophrenic fell while depressives concomitantly grew. The changes were related to a change from hospital to primary care base, indicating the importance of agency base.

Some studies have described or evaluated CPNs' work. Sladden's (1979) Edinburgh nurses worked primarily with women, unmarried and unemployed people. Their main problems were lack of social contacts, personality problems, family problems and difficulties with everyday activities. Some features of the clientele were apparently associated with specific nursing tasks, particularly phenothiazine injections for schizophrenic people. Clinical and psychosocial functions were by far the most frequently mentioned practice aims and methods; clinically oriented aims were associated with clinical attendance and psychosocial aims with community visits. However, while clinical functions were described in appropriate technical language, there was a lack of theoretical basis for interpersonal aspects of work, resulting in a difficulty defining needs and problems in ways which could be used for rational selection of methods. There was a tendency to refer environmental problems to social workers. Overall this indicated a frame of reference emphasizing a clinical perspective, concomitantly reducing attentiveness to social problems with which they had difficulty knowing how to deal. Hunter (1978) undertook a retrospective comparison of clients receiving a hospital based CPN service over five years with those not receiving such care. This service was associated with a greater number of hospital admissions where the reverse was hoped for, although fewer CPN than comparative group clients failed to take medication. Both groups had similar proportions in employment, and for a similar length of time, but social contacts were rather lower amongst the CPN group. Interviews with caregivers showed three quarters considered them helpful, with abilities to be friendly, understanding and liaise with doctors. However, only a fifth of the CPN and no comparative caregivers would turn first to CPNs for help, with an even lower figure for patients.

Paykel and Griffiths (1983) conducted a controlled trial comparing CPN work with chronic neurotic clients with outpatients receiving routine psychiatric after care, primarily using clinical and social adjustment measures. Mean symptom levels of both groups decreased over time, and although there was some intra group variability, differences between groups were slight and not significant. Social adjustments also showed some improvement but there were no significant differences between the two groups. Family burden ratings were obtained for a limited number of clients, but again there were no significant differences. They concluded that for all these ratings CPNs were as effective (or ineffective!) as routine psychiatric follow up. These results may be interesting compared with Corney's (1984a) a on c group. Some benefits were identified. Psychiatric outpatient visits were greatly reduced in the CPN group, and greater number of discharges were achieved without deleterious consequences. Most contacts were with the client alone and the most common activities identified were information and instruction, support/reassurance, ventilation and enhancement of self awareness. Patients' views showed a tendency for greater satisfaction with nurses who were considered more caring, easier to talk to, interested and more able to relax their clients. However, only half their clients saw them as the main treatment agent, whereas this was generally considered to be the psychiatrist in the outpatient group.

Marks and his colleagues (1977, 1985) have studied nurses as behaviour therapists. The first (1977) study was primarily hospital based, but showed improvement in phobic and obsessive compulsive disorders. The second (1985) control study examined neurotic clients in primary care settings in diagnostic areas most likely to respond to behavioural treatment (mainly phobics). Overall CPN clients improved significantly more than controls receiving GP care in most target behaviour areas and social adjustment. These are, of course, specialist nurses rather than CPNs, and strictly represent a vindication of psychological behavioural approaches rather than training general to CPNs. Skidmore and Friend (1984) who studied 1000 CPN visits to clients commented that 'community psychiatric nurses' work methods have developed more by trial and error than by logical progression' and cited their research showing little difference between those holding CPN post qualifying training and these without it. Indeed they found only 1 per cent of visits were for counselling.

Work has been published though only in article form (Wooff, 1988a and b) comparing CPNs and social workers in Salford. More detailed analysis is available from Wooff's PhD (1987). It was broadly divided into two. First, client diagnosis was examined through case register data, and is discussed above. CPNs tended to hold clients longer than social workers in continuous care. The second part was based on a study of face to face work with clients, involving ten CPNs and five social workers. She found CPNs and social workers gave similar amounts of support and advice, but social workers asked significantly more questions than CPNs and used general conversation less. Social workers were considerably more concerned with social adjustment than medical issues, while the reverse was the case for CPNs. Work largely reflected this: the main social work activities were counselling and practical assistance, while the main CPN activity was drug administration. Following client contact social workers were more likely to contact outside agencies. CPNs contacted each other or primary care professionals. This appeared related to work base. Overall Wooff attributed differences largely to theoretical base: with little theory of their own CPNs relied on a medical emphasis, while social workers possessed a psychosocial theory base. However, her cursory glance at theory provides little foundation for these comments.

The Study

The examination of professional and policy developments together with existing studies, demonstrates a great need for further research. In particular the development of community care, with CMHCs as a significant means for care delivery, the awareness of widespread minor mental illness in the general population, the potential significance of non-medical approaches to working with these problems and the competing role claims of CPNs and social workers present issues in urgent need of further examination. This book aims to do precisely that: it is a study and comparison of the theory and practice of social work and CPNs at a mental health centre. 'Theory' here refers to the knowledge and skills foundations for practice. It represents a number of advances on previous work.

1 There is currently no published research on the work of social workers and CPNs at CMHCs and in view of developments this research is of some importance.
2 The two occupations were based in the same agency and hence exposed to the same overall clientele. Agency function, as Wooff (1987) noted is significant. Her research examined social workers and CPNs in different settings, creating a further variable affecting comparison.
3 CMHCs have, as Sayce (1989) noted, tended to work with previously (specialist) untreated morbidity, usually managed in general practice and involving neurotic problems. Research offered the opportunity of examining specialist non-medical intervention with those previously without access to specialist help.

4 Decisions about who should do what were made in relation to the same overall pool of clients. It became possible thereby to examine the division of labour between CPNs and social workers.

Wooff's study, although providing welcome information, suffers two further disadvantages. Although she relates CPN-social work differences to the psychosocial theory base of social work compared with the lack of any substantive CPN theory and a consequent reliance on medical perspectives, she fails to examine in detail these theory bases. These, as we shall see, present very complex issues. Second, she consciously takes 'the perspective of community medicine'. This endows her research with meanings which may at times coincide with the professions studied, but which are, taken as a whole, external to them. Such external approaches, furthermore, evaluate the subjects in terms of the external agents — hence implicitly subordinating both CPNs and social workers to community medicine. Our research is characterized by three approaches.

1 A comparative analysis of theory, which provides the basis for practice.
2 A comparative analysis of the practice of CPNs and social workers, examining both division of labour and different approaches to intervention.
3 An examination of clients' views of intervention focusing particularly on agreement and disagreement with workers on perceptions of intervention, and their perception of workers' skills.

The examination of both theory *and* practice may help us judge the relative merits of the territorial claims of CPNs and social workers, and where their strengths and weaknesses lie. The former provides some indication of the knowledge and skills foundations while the latter examines the actual practice.

This study was based on the work of the Walk In Service (WIS), which took referrals from any community agency, professional or individual, at a CMHC in an urban setting in Southern England. This comprised one element of the community psychiatric facilities of the district. The city had a population of about 250,000 which was overwhelmingly white. The district was served by an old mental hospital which, like elsewhere, has in recent years combined a reduction in bed occupancy with increased resources in the community. Another community based unit contained social work, nurse behaviour therapist and outpatient services, in addition to which there was a drug-alcohol unit. The adult nursing service comprised behaviour therapy and rehabilitation teams (the latter associated with transferring long stay patients into community settings), an elderly care team and general psychiatry team. The general psychiatry team comprised eleven CPNs responsible to a senior CPN, and received referrals of those aged between 18 and 65 from various sources, particularly acute admissions wards, and increasingly from the WIS. The mental health social work team was part of the health district team of social services. It comprised one social work supervisor (senior) and nine social workers. The team carried both in patient and community based services. Areas of work included acute psychiatry, rehabilitation and elderly care. The general psychiatry CPN team and mental health social work team staffed the WIS. All the social workers were qualified and had a minimum of three years post qualifying experience in a mental health setting and all but one were approved under the Mental Health Act. All the CPNs involved held the RMN (Registered Mental Nurse) qualification and had extensive post qualification experience, the minimum being five years and the maximum twenty-eight years. With the exception of one CPN, they had worked in a community setting for at least three years, with most above five years. Most CPNs had taken post qualifying training, primarily developments in psychiatry, and a short course in behavioural work. None, however, had taken the post qualifying CPN training (English National Board, ENB 810, 811, 812). However, this was a stable team with extensive community experience. It is not clear that CPN training has an impact on practice (Reed, 1988), and the overwhelming majority of CPNs (four fifths) do not, in the most recent national survey (CPNA, 1985b) have this post qualifying training.

The CMHC was situated in a quiet road near the city centre with easy access from all parts of the city through public transport. The Centre provided out patient facilities, a day centre, psychological services and the WIS. The WIS was set up in 1978 and was one of the most well established community based services available directly to the public in Britain. It had a number of elements.

1 The provision of a specialist assessment and crisis intervention service.
2 A specialist advisory service to local agencies and professionals.
3 An easily accessible counselling service to clients and families.
4 Acting as specialist gatekeepers, assessing clients, and where appropriate referring them on to other agencies or professionals.

The service was established and primarily resourced by the mental health social work and general psychiatry CPN teams. Organization and planning were made by the senior CPN and social worker: it was *not*, therefore, headed by a psychiatrist and was very much a CPN-social work service. Additional medical input was provided by a psychiatric registrar. Referrals to the WIS represented, as noted earlier, one (important) source of social work and CPN work, although not all of them were involved. There was, furthermore, strong emphasis on what was perceived by workers as two related themes: joint work and role blurring. This was, it was felt, facilitated by shared office accommodation which helped interprofessional learning and the development of shared perspectives. The WIS pamphlet claimed (WIS, 1989) that the arrangement 'greatly reduces demarcation disputes and a considerable amount of learning and problem sharing takes place'.

The WIS operated a duty service each weekday from 9.00 am to 5.00 pm. At other times cover was provided by an out of hours social work team. Referrals were accepted from any source, and included a 'walk in' service for clients and their relatives. The duty team generally comprised a social worker, one or two CPNs, and the psychiatric registrar. The team endeavoured to undertake joint multiprofessional assessment, but the pressure of referral often made this impossible, and they might only be seen by one professional. Clients might be seen at home, or at the centre, or occasionally elsewhere. There were three likely outcomes. The client might be seen once or perhaps twice and no further intervention occurred. Alternatively, an assessment could be followed by referral on to other agencies or professionals (e.g. in-patient, behaviour therapy, district social services). Third, clients could be taken on by a CPN or social worker for short term or long term caseload intervention. This would occur at the allocation meeting attended by CPNs and social workers on Monday mornings.

The WIS possessed a number of characteristics sought by CMHCs. In terms of models identified (Sayce, 1987; Dick, 1985) it contained elements of two models: that where the CMHC acts as a 'funnel' through which clients are passed on to local resources, and that which offers specialist services such as counselling and groupwork. It emphasized also further elements: accessibility was stressed by the walk in service, its geographical availability, and its quick response to referrals. It involved multidisciplinary teamwork, without medical leadership encouraging greater interprofessional equality, and emphasized though not exclusively, a psychosocial approach. Finally, its gatekeeping element gave access to a comprehensive range of resources, and it had community links in terms of its relationship with health and social service agencies, although clients were not involved in managing service development.

Details about the conduct and timing of the study are given in Appendix 1. Chapter 2 examines the way in which social workers and CPNs define the phenomena with which they deal and the nature and scope of theory underlying practice. Chapters 3, 4 and 5 are based on a survey of the work of the WIS. Analysis is based on the framework provided in Chapter 2. Chapter 6 examines the interpersonal relationship practice foundations, Chapter 7 compares clients and workers' perceptions of intervention, and Chapters 8 and 9 discuss clients' perceptions of workers' skills. Chapter 10 concludes the study. We may first, then, turn to the theoretical base.

Theoretical Foundations

Nursing literature in particular has called for a more scientific professional base (Kim, 1983; Reihl and Roy, 1980) while social work has conducted a drive for an adequate research base (Davies, 1974). Such an enterprise is necessarily both conceptual and empirical — hence research developments must be founded on a clear conceptual framework (Harre, 1970; Keat and Urry, 1982). This chapter will outline a framework through which theory developments by both CPNs and social workers may be examined. The development of this framework is useful in itself for individual professions by identifying core elements of these professions. However, comparative analysis of two professions can highlight still more effectively these core elements. Finally, it can provide, by identifying key elements, the base for a more empirical, research based analysis of each profession's work.

There are two key elements to such conceptual developments. First we must work from meanings and expectations arising from within the professions themselves. What distinguishes professional actions is not just their concerns or behaviour, but the meanings attached to these by members of the profession (Kim, 1983; Rees, 1978). Hence we are concerned with what they think they are doing, who are their 'constituents', how they should work and so on. Second this must provide a basis for operational measurements which are applicable to practice, i.e. transfer the more theoretical considerations to practice work. This is no easy matter, and it becomes more difficult with two separate professions: we must provide a framework which is meaningful to both professions in order to compare them.

Our framework will be divided as follows:

1 Knowledge orientation
2 Practice orientation
3 Defining the client or patient
4 Context of intervention
5 Contexts specific to mental health
6 Direction of work with clients
7 Duration of intervention.

The analysis will conceptualize CPNs and mental health social workers as branches of their professions, i.e. emphasizing one to be a nurse and the other a social worker. Butterworth (1984) has suggested that CPNs and general nurses do not share common perspectives or roles. However, as will become apparent, CPNs have developed no distinctive theory of their own, and hence, unless they become something other than nurses, are reliant on the theory base commonly shared amongst nurses.

Knowledge Orientation

Social work has, for some considerable time, emphasized its social science knowledge base (Leonard 1975, Bartlett 1970). This social science emphasis produces predefined categories — stigma, class, socialization, attachment etc. — which provide a means for interpreting situations through a range of alternative explanations. Hence child battering may occur through stress, failure of attachment, poverty, cycle of abuse and so on (Sheppard, 1982). They provide *reasons* or *causes* for what is occurring, thus making clients' actions meaningful.

These explanations occur within broad paradigms, of which Leonard (1975) identifies two: physical science and human science, each of which have further subdivisions according to emphasis within these paradigms. These paradigms to a considerable degree involve commitment to different knowledge assumptions, hence even within social science controversy exists about how to interpret and resolve particular problems. However, this largely exclusive use of social science knowledge may exclude consideration of alternative knowledge domains. Those derived from physiology or biology, for example — if not literally unthinkable because of the 'seepage' from alternative disciplines in everyday life (e.g. through the media or visiting the doctor) — will nonetheless in practice be minimized in importance. The interpretive frameworks in the form of 'legitimate professional knowledge' will both emphasize social science knowledge and de-legitimate alternatives. Hence explanations of depression emphasizing social deprivation and feminist perspectives will have more influence on social work than biological explanations, particularly when compared with the medical profession (Corob, 1987).

However, there is no unified professional view of the place of social science knowledge — an illustration of professional segmentation (Bucher and Strauss, 1966). Some — although a small minority — have sought to marginalize social science. Davies (1986) suggests that social science has done little to improve practice, while Howe (1980) argues that it is riven by such great paradigmatic and theoretical disputes as to make it difficult to develop a knowledge base or apply it with any effectiveness. Others, however, accept the necessity of social science, seeking to identify means for choosing and applying appropriate approaches. Stevenson (1971) suggests 'frames of reference' by which a range of available theoretical contributions may be examined in specific practice contexts. Others are concerned that eclecticism provides no route to an adequate knowledge base. Sheldon (1978) argues for the need to develop a common perspective on evidence — criteria which are scientific (emphasizing refutability) and by which some knowledge may be adopted and other knowledge discarded. Sheppard (1984) suggests choice of knowledge for any particular problem should be based on explanatory adequacy — measured in terms of values, theoretical framework, methodology and consistency of findings — and its applicability in practice. Despite Davies' criticisms, and although debate exists about *how* it should be applied, social science remains the dominant knowledge base for social work. Indeed, Hardiker (1981) maintains it is indispensable, drawing on research to demonstrate that it makes the difference between adequate practice and possible disasters.

The presentation of the CPN knowledge base is different in a number of respects. Reflecting professional role, knowledge focuses specifically on mental health. Although there is some variation (Davis, 1986, Kalkman and Davis, 1974) this is generally organized in terms of models or psychiatric ideologies. Hence Burgess, A. (1985) states:

> the specific tasks and activities used in psychiatric nursing are best described within ... conceptual models of psychiatric mental health care

a view with which others concur (Carr *et al.*, 1980; Stuart and Sundeen, 1983; Mitchell, 1974; Puttnam, 1981). Two reasons for their significance are presented: constructing a model of mental illness allows us to see its nature, causation and effects (Mitchell, 1974), and they allow nurses to function rationally and evaluate their effectiveness (Stuart and Sundeen, 1983). Because they go beyond social science this represents a broader trawling of knowledge but with a narrower focus (mental health) than evident in social work. The use of models is allied to the general advocacy of eclecticism. It is seen as a means of overcoming the 'limitations' and 'simplifications' of theory, and the belief that there is no 'right way' to approach problems (Lancaster, 1980). Neither eclecticism nor the choice of model is generally seen as problematic — choice may be based on the nurse's personal preference, provided it is explicit (Burgess, 1985). Although some social workers also advocate eclecticism (Pincus and Minahan, 1975; Whittaker, 1974), they appear more aware of inherent inconsistencies, the threat to developing a consistent knowledge base and the need for rigorous criteria to choose between models. 'The nursing literature' writes Sladden 'does not waste time over the conceptual problems of the eclectic approach' (1979).

The delineation of models reflects an awareness of their interest to psychiatry as a whole (Siegler and Osmond, 1966; Strauss *et al.*, 1964; Tyrer and Steinberg, 1987). Model construction, however, varies between different authors. The core division, identifying medical, social and psychological models, is presented by Mitchell (1974). The medical model (Burgess calls this 'biologic'), he says, presents psychiatric disorder like any other involving a pathological lesion and disturbed function which is resolved physiologically (e.g. by drugs). Others add a characteristic process of examination, diagnosis, treatment and prognosis (Carr *et al.*, 1980; Stuart and Sundeen, 1983). Mitchell suggests the social model focuses on individuals' failure to function in groups, while others emphasize the causal significance of social environment and conditions. The third model is psychological, which is presented as behavioural disturbance or distress due to powerful psychological forces, resolved only by therapy confronting the intra-psychic conflicts. However, additional divisions exist between psychoanalytic and behavioural or cognitive behavioural models (Burgess, 1985; Stuart and Sundeen, 1983), and 'Third Force' psychology emphasizing peoples' potential for personal growth. Stuart and Sundeen (1983) present two further models, existential and interpersonal, emphasizing the importance of relations *between* people. A 'community orientation', loosely defined as an ideology focusing on those needing help but unwilling or unable to seek it, is identified by Carr *et al.* (1980) (*cf.* Baker and Schulberg, 1967). Finally Davey (1984) identifies an anti-psychiatry perspective (better called perspectives) broadly denying the validity of an illness label for those suffering psychiatric problems. Overall, although models may be helpful, the CPN is confronted by a great, perhaps bewildering, variety of alternatives and no consensus about divisions between them.[1]

Practice Orientation: Judgment and Experience

The limited nature of social science knowledge concomitantly increases the importance of judgment and experience, well recognized in social work. Emphasizing the importance of judgment, Howe (1980) states it

> cannot be resolved into information and documented in the way information can ... for some skills judgment may form the greater part of their knowledge.

while Sheppard (1984) suggests:

> it is often easier to identify the uniqueness of and differences between one person and another ... many studies are too general to provide a clear direction to practitioners working with specific problems and clients.

Indeed, those who emphasize social work as 'art' rather than 'technique' stress this most strongly. What is important in the process of social work, and what is effective in achieving its ends, they argue, is not some technical expertise, but the quality of the person of the helper (Jordan, 1979; Keith-Lucas, 1972). To a considerable degree this emphasizes the understanding of others by social workers: using abilities which most of us possess, but the social worker — to be any good — should develop to an advanced level.

> The worker knows about the client's meaning because of the worker's own 'human nature' tells him what it is to experience . . . mental or emotional states and can sensitively extrapolate from them. (England, 1986).

Additionally, their work leads to contact with problems to a far greater degree than normal social life, and involves focusing on these problems. Hence practice experience allows them to refine their understanding and responses to these problems, thus providing a legitimate 'knowledge base' in itself.

The issue of judgment is significant for nursing as a whole and CPNs in particular, though not all are agreed. Neuman (1980) and Johnson (1980) both emphasize the technical expertise derived from their models. Orem (1980) however, stressing personal qualities, recognizes the importance of particular techniques, but emphasizes the individual patient and correct nursing judgments. Most significant for good judgment is the nurse's experience, but other factors such as innate ability, life experience, personality and style of thinking are also important. Rogers (1970) also sees a relationship between the technical aspects of knowledge and the more creative, individualized, and experience based use of judgment in applying that knowledge:

> It must be thoroughly understood [she says] that tools and procedures are adjuncts to practice and are safe and meaningful only to the extent that knowledgeable nursing judgments underwrite their selection . . . [and] use.

These views, general to nursing, are apparent in psychiatric nursing. Hence Ward (1985) believes that:

> The nature of nursing . . . decreed that innate artistic qualities of human caring . . . should be incorporated into the general pattern.

Likewise, Barker (1985) states:

> Judgments . . . are found in almost all forms of patient care. Even when we use highly objective means of recording and measuring the patient's state . . . we end up using our own subjective judgments.

It is, then, as with social work, the limitations of knowledge when applied to practice which leaves experience and judgment a vital place in practice. Lack of experience and good judgment can be inimical to adequate practice. Kim (1983) writes

> Wrong decisions are made because the nurse has a limited experience of specific life and nursing situations with which he or she can develop evaluative framework.

In theoretical terms, judgments and experience are significant because they limit the effect on behaviour of knowledge approaches discrete to each profession. Of course, experience is not somehow divorced from theory — implicitly or explicitly used to give situations meaning. However, the more important experience is, the more scope exists for creative understanding and responses to problems on the part of individual practitioners. Indeed, where frequent contact occurs, this may well encourage 'seepage' of concepts and theories from one discipline to another.

Defining the Client or Patient

Both social workers and CPNs define clients with meanings particular to their profession: either in terms of problems or needs. Social workers' concern is with *psychosocial* problems or needs (Haines, 1981; Roberts and Nee, 1970). Reid (1978) refers to 'problem oriented theory' and states that the

> major concern of clinical social work is to alleviate problems of individuals and families.

Hoghughi (1980) also emphasizes problems, referring to the 'symbiotic relationship' of social work with social problems. 'Social work' he says, echoing Perlman (1957) 'is about solving problems.' Reid (1978) distinguished between *acknowledged* problems — problems clients consider themselves to have — and *attributed* problems — problems attributed by others, in this case social workers, to clients. Furthermore, fundamental disagreements exist about problem definition. What does or does not constitute a social problem depends upon the social processes by which it becomes a matter of concern as well as theoretical assumptions underlying them (Rubington and Weinberg, 1977). Social work definitions of problems possess implicit standards influenced greatly by their position in Social Service Departments (Howe, 1979).

Need definitions also possess an ideological dimension. Hardiker, (1981; *cf.* Davies, 1982) argues that

> The social worker's brief in welfare states is to identify and meet personal need and find acceptable ways of representing deviants to the rest of society.

Their freedom to define need, however, she considers is limited by structural boundaries provided by their agency. Smith and Harris (1972), like other authors, argue that social workers adopt ideologies of need, based on perceptions of unit of need, cause of need and assessor of need. Rees (1978) indicates these ideologies are related closely to perceptions of moral character, while Hardiker (1977) suggests they are key to understanding central issues of punishment/freewill and treatment/determinism, and that interpretations of need are made through frameworks originating from psychological or sociological knowledge.

Nursing differs from social work in its emphasis on health. Their bio-psychosocial orientation is more ambitious than that of social work, which emphasizes only the psychosocial (Kim, 1983; Chrisman and Fowler, 1980, Pearson and Vaughn, 1984; Roper *et al.*, 1980; Kyes and Hofling, 1980). Kim (1983) argues that problem or need definition is critical for nursing diagnosis, providing a means for conceptualizing the client in terms of the concerns of nursing. Both Henderson (1964) and Roper *et al.* (1981) perceive need as nurses' central concern: they are interested in the 'observable behavioural manifestations of basic human needs' (Roper *et al.*, 1980). This is just as true for CPNs: Simmons and Brooker (1986) state that 'true mental health requires basic needs are met.' Likewise Carr *et al.* (1980) suggest that 'patients need to be approached as individuals who have needs.' However, when need is explored more deeply, there is little reference to its ideological component. Maslow's hierarchy of need — which is, like other need definitions, ideological — is particularly influential (Maslow, 1970). This hierarchy of need has five levels from basic physiological needs through more 'advanced' needs up to self actualization. These are ordered in priority: it is only when the lower needs are satisfied that motivation is established to seek fulfilment of higher level needs.

Nursing is also conceived in terms of problems. Rambo (1984) indeed recognizes the relevance of both need and problem definition, but suggests the superiority of the latter by linking it with scientificity. 'The nursing process' she writes 'as a method of problem solving represents a scientific avenue of nursing care.' Barker (1985) likewise prefers problem identification to (medical) diagnosis in psychiatric nursing.

> The common denominator [he suggests] is the search for and ultimate detection of, problems.... Aspects of a person's performance and presentation which might be ignored or overlooked in (medical) diagnosis will be caught under this broader frame of reference.

Problem definition in nursing, however, must reflect nursing's concern with the biopsychosocial aspects of the human condition. Stevens (1979), for example, lists five conditions: experiential states, physiological deviations, problematic behaviour, altered relationships and reactions of others. However, problem identification is largely theory related — hence different approaches will emphasize different aspects (Roy and Roberts, 1981; Orem, 1980). Nonetheless, problem identification is seen as crucial to the development of a nursing classification system — it becomes a tool for intervention (Roy, 1975): 'an essential next step in the development of the science of nursing.' What is required is not a problem classification which is atheoretical — which is not possible — but one which is framed in terms of meanings appropriate to CPNs (and social workers) and which may be applied across different models (Kim, 1983). Kim suggests problem identification requires three elements: a problem label, a definition of causal elements, and a description of the characteristics of the phenomenon, interestingly close to that advocated by Huntington (1981) for social work.

Context for Intervention

The context of social work practice, like problem definition, reflects its psychosocial orientation and the related intervention modes. Social work possesses theoretical diversity and some conflicting assumptions. Practice is rarely characterized by explicit use of theory, but when examined closely, theoretical constructs provide an implicit though critical context for practice. Curnock and Hardiker (1979) have shown that good practice requires theory, without which mistakes would be made. It necessarily involves flexible and imaginative use of such theory. However, because of this theoretical diversity it is difficult to characterize social work in terms of a particular approach: it is best reflected in the pragmatic use of different contexts for intervention rather than specific methods which may be adopted. Analysis based on a specific method would not reflect the known, and diverse, use of theory in practice.

Recent theoretical developments suggest four stages. The basic division is between interpersonal intervention, largely but not exclusively concerned with clients, and environmental intervention, involving individuals and systems within the social structure in the process of providing services to the client (Haines, 1981). This configuration, classically presented by Hollis (1972) was 'person in situation': the person, his situation and the interaction between them. She referred to 'internal' and 'external' pressure to signify forces within the individual and the environment. Drawing on psychoanalytic and sociological concepts, intervention involved addressing both internal psychological conflicts and 'life pressures' such as economic deprivation, poor housing and educational disadvantage. Bartlett's (1970) concern with social work's overemphasis on the client's immediate circumstances led to her conception of 'interventive repertoire', involving the use of a variety of approaches as appropriate. Hence the practitioners may involve themselves with the client, encourage groups, develop social supports and act for change within the community. Work could be both proactive and reactive. Unitary models attempted to provide a conceptual schema for this repertoire, moving beyond a 'dichotomous view' of people and environment, to a focus on linkages between people and resource systems (Pincus and Minahan, 1975). This systems approach meant the issue was not:

> who has the problem, but how the elements of the situation ... are interacting to frustrate people coping with their tasks.

The ecological perspective has much in common with unitary models. However, it goes one stage further by identifying 'levels' of context. Whittaker and Garbarino (1983) developed a four-fold distinction based on concepts of social networks and support. To a considerable degree this provides a theoretical base for community social work developments (NISW, 1982). Microsystems represent the immediate social networks of individuals — their family, school, immediate workplace and so on. Mesosystems are the relationships *between* these microsystems (e.g. relations between home, school and work related groups). Exosystems are situations that affect a person's development, but in which the person does not play a direct role. These include political agencies and centres of economic influence. Macrosystems are ideological and cultural expectations in a society: they reflect shared beliefs creating behavioural patterns (e.g. how cultures define and respond to dependency, how political ideologies allocate resources between public and private agencies and different groups). Whittaker (1974) calls work using this ecological approach social treatment. He defines five major roles (Whittaker, 1986):

1 Treatment agent
2 Teacher — counsellor
3 Broker of services or resources
4 Advocate
5 Network/systems consultant

Each of these represent role clusters — ways of working or responsibilities the professional may assume according to the circumstances of the case and may operate in different and overlapping contexts.

Wooff (1987) suggests community psychiatric nursing is characterized by the lack of a theoretical base:

> Neither psychiatric nurses nor CPNs have developed a common set of principles or an organized set of professional values ... integral ... for decision making skills.

However, models exist in the wider realm of nursing as a whole. In this respect it resembles social work — possessing models which are, on the whole, general to the profession but not specific to psychiatry. Kim (1983) classifies nursing in terms of its domain. Using Kim, we can distinguish two areas in the *domain* of nursing — the phenomena with which it is concerned

— that focusing on the patient and that focusing on the environment. Beyond Kim's typology, however, we can distinguish the *context* of nursing — the phenomena on which it will act — from its domain. This likewise can be divided between client and environment.

Although a variety of different approaches are available — activities of living, interpersonal, total person, behavioural systems and so on — two broad factors are consistent to these models. First nursing concerns itself with biopsychosocial factors affecting health. Hence Kim (1983) writes:

> the nursing perspective is to conceptualize a person as a biopsycho-social being with an emphasis on health.

a position adopted by other theorists (Roy, 1976; Neuman, 1982; Rogers, 1970). This is both all embracing in terms of the human condition and more ambitious than the more limited psychosocial concerns of social work. Second, while the *domains* of interest to nursing frequently encompass bio-psychosocial aspects of both patient and environment, the *context* of intervention invariably focuses primarily on the patient. This can at times appear as a puzzling disjunction, between domains relevant to health, such as social factors which suggest the need for environmental intervention, and the specific intervention focus on the patient. This may be related to perceptions of the appropriate role of the nurse, which would lead to the development of role appropriate models for practice. This individualism is consistent with some models emphasizing nurse-patient interaction. King's (1981) theory of goal attainment emphasizes interactional elements — particularly 'nurse-client interactions that lead to achievement of goals.' She is quite explicit: although the domains of concern for nursing are personal, interpersonal and social systems, and health problems may be caused by environmental stress, the main focus for action is the nurse-patient dyad. Others claim domains which are equally comprehensive, without being explicit as King is, about the narrower focus for intervention. Rogers' (1970) concept of Unitary Man accepts only the inter-connectedness, *in reality*, of environmental and human elements, although conceding the possibility of distinguishing *conceptually* between the two. Johnson's model (Johnson, 1980; Grubb, 1980) recognizes physical, psychological and social elements, and expresses interest in the domains of both client and environment. Grubb (1980) lists a number of relevant environmental variables, yet: 'The predominant focus of nursing is on the person who is ill or threatened with illness.' Roy also recognizes both personal and environmental variables, with physiological, self concept, role function and interdependence elements (Roy and Roberts, 1981). She, however, emphasizes the need for individual adaptation to the environment whether involving biophysical or social elements. This, of course, begs the question: just how adequate for health is the environment to which the patient must adapt?

This disjunction between domain and context is well illustrated by

Rambo's (1984) explication of Roy's model. She clearly recognizes many American black peoples' health is affected by structural disadvantage, involving segregation, discrimination and poverty. She also recognizes these can affect the patient's health and performance, causing maladaptive behaviour, with which the nurse is legitimately concerned. Yet the nurse should only work with the patient to:

> attempt to bring *their* [my italics] maladaptive behaviour within the normal or adaptive range.

There is no concern here to work on those environmental factors *directly* which cause large numbers of black people ill health.

Some writers do recognize approaches beyond the individual, although they are more tentative and lack the alternatives available to social work. Kim (1983) differentiates between the client-nurse system, involving nurse-patient interaction, and the nurse system, largely excluding the patient, but does little more. Pepleau, whose interest is primarily in a therapeutic interpersonal process does advocate involvement in health care planning and social policy issues (Pepleau, 1962, 1980). However, between individual work and social policy issues, she has little on work with patients in an environmental context. Neuman (1982) goes further in this direction. She recognizes nurses' claim to be concerned with phenomena relating to both client and environment. She identifies stressors originating in intrapersonal, interpersonal and extrapersonal areas. Additionally, however, she suggests preventive care and health education programmes, and that nurses should help 'individuals, families and groups' attain a maximum level of wellness (Neuman, 1980). Chapman (1985) suggests this model is useful applied not just to individuals but also communities.

This dominant individualist focus — contrasting with detailed theoretical developments beyond individual clients in social work — is significant because, as Kim (1983) suggests, the focus provides a 'space' within which knowledge and skills may develop. A dominant individualism militates against the inclusion of skills oriented to the environment in the nurse's repertoire.

Contexts Specific to Mental Health

Social work approaches to mental health problems largely entail the application of their broader professional skills to the more specific area of mental health. As with other areas of work such as child care, they limit their concern — wide enough in itself — to the psychosocial, perceived to complement the more biophysical medical orientation of psychiatrists. This approach is supported by social psychiatry research which has emphasized the interconnection between those very personal and environmental factors on which social work skills concentrate (Cochrane, 1983; Miles, 1987). Much of the social work knowledge development specific to psychiatry involves identification and recognition of mental disorders, core — in more detail — to psychiatric nurse training, examining this in terms of the social process, context and prognosis of mental illness (Hudson, 1982; Munro and McCulloch, 1969; Butler and Pritchard, 1983). In recent years, Approved Social Work training has emphasized the legal context as well as symptom recognition plus specific skills in case material analysis (Central Council for Education and Training in Social Work [CCETSW], 1986).

The theoretical limits of nursing as a whole clearly disadvantage CPNs interested in placing patients within a broader environmental context. Developments in this respect specific to CPNs are extremely recent. Moore commented when introducing one significant book in 1980 (Carr *et al.*, 1980) that it was: 'but a starting point in the debate on community psychiatric nursing.' Another writer (Ward, 1985) stated that:

> there are very few texts available to United Kingdom nurses which relate ... to the very special needs ... of psychiatry.

Indeed, the community rather than institutional hospital perspective has led to an emphasis on individualized care of the patient (Carr *et al.*, 1980; Ward, 1985). Some attempts to incorporate a psychosocial dimension have not transcended this individualism. Hence Barry (1984) developing Roy's adaptation model focuses on the patient, emphasizing psychological rather than social variables. Likewise Barker (1985) emphasizes a 'person centred approach' designed to identify what is significant for 'this particular patient' who is 'a unique person.'

In the face of theoretical limitations, CPNs have, to a considerable degree, taken refuge in skills information, pragmatically chosen on the basis of professional need (Marram, 1973; Looms and Horsley, 1974). This is largely 'borrowed' knowledge, generated within other disciplines, but apparently useful to CPNs. Barker (1985) states, for example, that

> The methods I discuss in this book are influenced strongly by psychological research and practice.

In this respect, approaches like social skills, and particularly behaviourism have taken on some significance (Roach and Farley, 1986; Marks *et al.*, 1977; Barker, 1982; Pope, 1986; Hargie and McCarton, 1986). Given the psychological orientation, the focus tends primarily to be on the individual, although there is a greater interest in their immediate interactional context, as with behavioural approaches. Likewise, Pope (1986) discusses family skills training in relation to high expressed emotion families of schizophrenic patients.

A potentially wider context is provided by an ecological approach (Lancaster, 1980) emphasizing the:

> dynamic interaction between the patient's internal environment and the multiple external environments.

These are linked by a systems approach, but there is little theoretical development, such as different types and levels of environmental intervention. Rather, there are hints of relevant factors such as familial or social systems linkages, which are not fully developed. The exploration of the context of social environment has been rather too brief for detailed skills development (Carr *et al.*, 1980). Simmons and Brooker (1986) have been boldest in this respect, examining in some detail social factors in the family and wider society. Their analysis is stimulating, suggesting wider possible contexts for intervention, but ultimately limited in detail about the ways to work in these wider social contexts. Overall, then, while nursing does possess a theoretical base, CPNs may be viewed as struggling to free themselves from its limits. They have taken a few tentative steps without developing a consistent theoretical base beyond individualism.

Direction of Work with Clients

The client/environment distinction relevant to both social work and nursing may be related to direct and indirect work. This is a distinction extensively used in social work as a means of delineating the locus of intervention (Specht and Vickery, 1978; Whittaker, 1974; Haines, 1981; Whittaker and Garbarino, 1983). In our framework it is significant because it indicates the worker's approach to particular problems, hence linking problem type with locus of intervention. Whittaker (1974) adopts the most frequently used definitions. Direct work is 'what the worker does directly in their face to face encounter.' Indirect helping 'refers to all activities that the worker undertakes on behalf of the client to further mutually agreed upon goals' i.e. work with others designed to influence the client's behaviour and/or circumstances. Middleman and Goldberg (1974) extend this to a second category — the problem group. Hence working with people with common problems — e.g. schizophrenic people or those in poverty — constitutes direct work. Working with others concerned with that problem — agencies, voluntary organizations, even politicians — constitutes indirect work. Specht and Vickery (1978) identify two further uses of the term. In relation to groupwork, attempts to influence an individual directly are contrasted with work on the structural relations of the group or others in the group, which is indirect. Finally, it may relate to the *participation* of the worker in problem solving. Direct work entails actual involvement with the client in problem solving. Indirect work involves discussing the relevant problem with the client, without the worker being present when the problem is actually worked upon. For our purposes, the most frequently used distinction — that of Whittaker — is most helpful. It can be as easily applied to CPNs as social workers, and is relevant to problems. Specht and Vickery (1978) argue this is most appropriate — whether an approach is direct or indirect, the *focus* is on the particular problem with which client and worker are concerned.

Duration of Intervention

The final element is the duration of intervention. This issue has been particularly prominent in social work, although because some of the approaches used transcend that particular occupation — e.g. crisis intervention, psychoanalytically and behaviorally oriented methods — the debate has considerable relevance for CPNs. Perlman (1969) commented on a previously well established tendency by social workers to value longer term work without, compared with brief work, demonstrating its greater effectiveness. Extended work is associated with three general influences. Psychoanalysis has influenced significantly the knowledge base of social work. With its emphasis on in-depth analysis of underlying psychological problems, and development of 'insight' (a term used by social workers differently from psychoanalysts) it has a tendency towards lengthy intervention (Yelloly, 1980; Hollis, 1972). Others regard the 'relationship' as crucial. By valuing relationships for their own sake, and where the goal is presented as self realization or self-fulfilment, importance is implicitly attached to extended intervention (Keith-Lucas, 1972; Jordan, 1979). Although an end in itself, the relationship is also seen as the most effective means of promoting change (Truax and Carkhuff, 1967). A third associated element is a generalized 'supportive' orientation of some social workers. In mental health work, the professional role becomes a form of 'unlimited supportive friendship' coupled with practical help. Additionally there is little negotiation of the purpose of the work if this places the 'friendship' in jeopardy (Fisher *et al.*, 1984).

Extended intervention may be long term by design, but tends instead to be 'open ended' rather than time limited. It may be of low or high intensity. However, advocates of brief intervention (Reid and Epstein, 1972): 'take the position that planned short term treatment should be the dominant form of contact.' Brief intervention is associated with task centred, crisis intervention and some behavioural work (Reid, 1978; Rappaport, 1970; Sheldon, 1982). Crisis intervention emphasizes the therapeutic potential of work over a relatively short crisis period (Rappaport, 1970). During this period the client is in a state of disequilibrium, when normal problem solving techniques are ineffective. However, there are natural processes of growth and development which, during this time, the worker may help mobilize in the client. Key characteristics of this approach are that it is both goal oriented and time limited, in this respect similar to task centred work. This also emphasizes exactitude in formulating problems, methods to deal with them, and evaluation of outcome. Task centred work is more widely applicable, not limited to states of crisis. Rather than emphasizing in-depth work (or 'underlying conditions') task centred work directs change efforts at *manifest* problems of interpersonal conflict — role performance and the like — working on the 'here and now'. Although there is an element of expediency in advocating brief intervention (given limited resources) supporters argue it is no less effective than extended work (Reid, 1978). Some intervention is unintentionally brief because clients discontinue contact, but debates on duration reflect basic differences in philosophies of practice.

Concluding Comments

Social workers and CPNs have carried out a discourse about their respective occupations largely independent of each other. Comparison is instructive, providing a yardstick by which professional ideas and development may be measured against each other. The adequacy of the social work knowledge base, for example, is more realistically assessed when compared with the problems confronted by other occupations in developing and applying their own knowledge than when measured against some arbitary and perhaps ideal criteria (Howe, 1980). Although neither social work nor CPNs are rigidly demarked by approaches discrete to each profession they are characterized by significant differences of emphasis. Each is characterized by different elements (and degrees) of integration. Thus the biopsychosocial CPN orientation adopts models from wider realms of knowledge, but this is far from systematic lacking criteria for integration. Problems of eclecticism arise which are not confronted. Social work, with a less ambitious psychosocial orientation, has considered issues of integration within their narrower social science framework (Sheldon, 1978; Sheppard, 1984; Stevenson, 1971; Whittaker and Garbarino, 1983). Both professions, furthermore, recognize a significant degree of indetermination, hence the importance of judgment. When combined with paradigmatic and knowledge realm diversity, this indeterminacy encourages segmentation within these professions, with individuals or groups committed to different approaches. There is, furthermore, some overlap between these professions. Hence the uncertainty of the social science foundations of social work is reflected in the variety of available mental health models; significance is ascribed by both professions to judgment; both claim an interest in the psychosocial (though CPNs are also interested in the 'bio'); and both borrow knowledge from other disciplines, although unlike CPNs social workers have also generated their own knowledge (e.g. task centred, problem solving).

However, significant differences exist. Some issues of relevance to both professions, such as the duration of intervention, have been considered in detail only by social work. Phenomena are defined by CPNs through mental health models, and by social workers through their social science knowledge base. CPNs' theoretical base is more individualistic and far less well developed than social work. At the same time they claim a domain — biopsychosocial — far wider than that of social work. To a considerable degree this means they raise problems — such as the social disadvantage-illness relationship — with which their theory (or models) does not equip them to deal. We might suggest that CPNs make greater claims than social work but have less ability to 'deliver the goods'. It is possible to examine whether this, in fact, happens in practice. We may, furthermore, suggest three possible alternatives for a relationship between theory and practice. First, the discreteness of knowledge: the more each profession has a knowledge base discrete to itself, the greater the expected difference in behaviour between the two professions. Second, the knowledge base may be uncertain, and judgment may as a result play a significant part (indeterminate). The more indeterminate it is, the less the knowledge base differences may matter. Third, where close contacts exist between the professions, we may expect shared experience and negotiation of meanings would encourage mutual learning and increased similarities in behaviour (depending on the degree of knowledge indeterminancy). The three alternatives will be examined in the analysis of practice. However, before we do this it is necessary briefly to examine the work context provided by the agency.

Note

1 Mental health models and social science reflects the terms of discourse for social work and CPN knowledge. This does not prevent social workers from considering mental health models (much discussed by social scientists) or CPNs from considering social service influences on mental health models.

Chapter 3

Agency Work

The work of the WIS was examined through a survey of referrals. The survey, lasting four months showed 388 clients referred, of which a quarter (eighty) were not seen. Over 70 per cent of referrals were made by GPs (33 per cent) the client (27 per cent) or relatives, friends and acquaintances (11 per cent). This shows an emphasis on both primary care and direct referrals. In the latter respect they performed markedly better than the Lewisham Centre (Boardman *et al.*, 1987), indicating a more successful walk-in and self referral performance. Althogether nearly 85 per cent of referrals came from the general population or community agencies and professionals. Slightly over half (51 per cent) of clients referred were male, and two thirds were aged 20 to 44. The former figure is perhaps surprising in view of the excess of women over men suffering neurotic problems in general population studies. They tended to lack close social support: only 36 per cent were married (compared with three fifths in the general population), and a further 9 per cent were cohabiting. Only a third of clients, compared with 57 per cent of the local population were owner occupiers while those in council tenancies (30 per cent) was roughly equal. A third of clients, compared with 15 per cent of the local population were in private rented, lodging, hostel accommodation or no fixed abode. Over half the clients (53 per cent) were unemployed or in families with no employed member. Over three fifths of all referrals (61 per cent) relied on state benefit, not including child benefit. Over two thirds of those employed were in social class 3 or below. The clients referred, therefore, were grossly disadvantaged in a number of ways. They were less likely to be in a relationship where a partner offered close emotional support, they were less likely to be employed, or if employed below social class 2 and likely to be reliant on state benefit indicating low income. Their housing tenure was less secure than the general population, and many suffered multiple disadvantage.

While nearly two fifths of clients were self/relative/acquaintance referred there was further evidence of reaching those not otherwise receiving help. Three fifths (61 per cent) of clients were not currently receiving social service or psychiatric support, and for 38 per cent of clients, referral was their first

Table 3.1 Allocation

Social Workers	67 (21.8%)	Doctor	53 (17.2%)
CPN	62 (20.1%)	Doctor plus CPN	
CPN and social workers	71 (23.1%)	and/or social worker	55 (17.8%)

contact with psychiatric services. The main requests by referrers were for assessment (39 per cent), advice (18 per cent) counselling/emotional support (18 per cent) and hospital admission (15 per cent). These requests emphasize the importance of the specialist assessment service, while hospital admission requests also show the significance of the connection between community and hospital facilities.

All but a minority of clients were seen by a CPN or social worker, although the doctor played a significant part. The concept of primary problem was used to identify which, from among the psychiatric and social and health problems of clients, the workers considered most important. It provided a means, therefore, for some kind of central 'definition of the client' (see note 1, page 55). Overall 170 (55 per cent) clients were mental health cases, and 138 (43 per cent) had social or physical health primary problems (only 1 per cent had physical health primary problems). The largest groups were emotional and relationship problems (38 per cent), neurotic problems and personality disorders (28 per cent), psychotic (16 per cent), and drug or alcohol abuse (11 per cent). This demonstrates, first, how frequently clients were *not* seen primarily to suffer mental health problems, and second, the large swathe of neurotic, emotional and ·relationship problems. However, it is also noticeable that a sizeable minority had psychotic primary problems, reflecting, in part, the crisis service. Mental health problems were identified in 75 per cent of cases, emphasizing that they were present even where the primary problem was defined as social. However, 25 per cent did not have mental health problems, and over half of mental disorders identified (55 per cent) were defined as borderline cases. Depression was the most predominant of mental disorders comprising a fifth of all clients and 30 per cent of those with mental disorders. Anxiety and alcohol abuse each accounted for just over 10 per cent of clients. Social and physical health problems were broadly divided into three: practical, emotional and relationship and ill health. Over four fifths of clients (83 per cent) suffered at least one emotional or relationship problem. Practical problems occurred in 44 per cent of cases, while ill health affected a sizeable minority (24 per cent) of clients. More detailed classification showed nearly three fifths suffered emotional problems, 44 per cent had problems with social relations or isolation, 30 per cent had marital or cohabitee problems (i.e. most of those married or cohabiting!), and a fifth had problems of loss or separation. A high proportion of these clients, therefore, expressed profound problems with their social network, an issue frequently associated with mental health problems (Henderson *et al.*, 1981). Over a fifth

Table 3.2   Case Status

Brief Work	235 (76%)
Allocated and not seen	16 (5%)
Short/long term caseload	42 (14%)
Medical Allocation	15 (5%)

of clients had respectively financial and employment problems, and a quarter (24 per cent) had housing problems. About a sixth (18 per cent) of clients suffered minor physical ill health and 7 per cent had major ill health.

The proportion receiving brief (usually less than a week) intervention appears surprising (table 3.2). It may in part reflect immediate crisis help enabling the client. However, it mainly reflects their gatekeeping (assessment and disposal) role: 181 (72 per cent of brief clients) were referred to other agencies. One fifth of clients referred on became psychiatric in patients and a further 22 per cent were referred for outpatient treatment; 14 per cent went to GPs and 12 per cent to social services, while nearly a tenth went to a psychologist or CPN (either rehabilitation or behaviour therapy). Assessment and exploration of clients' problems occurred in 50 per cent of cases, while a further 12 per cent involved more specific mental health section assessments. This suggests detailed exploration of client problems may not always be necessary, perhaps because their problems were at times obvious or because the person was previously known and hence such detail was unnecessary. Discussing future options with clients occurred in 61 per cent of cases as was information and advice in 54 per cent. Emotional support or ventilation occurred with 34 per cent of clients. Practical resources were mobilized in 15 per cent of cases and drug treatment occurred with one tenth of clients.

Overall, then, the service was characterized by a number of elements. They possessed a very socially disadvantaged client group, consistent with research on the relation of disadvantage and mental health problems in the community (Cochrane, 1983). Referrals showed extensive community access (from GP, self/relatives and acquaintance referrals) and they also tapped a significant proportion of clients not previously subject to psychiatric help. Intervention showed three fifths of clients received joint multiprofessional help, and that the gatekeeping role, referring on to a spectrum of agencies and professionals was significant. Only a minority of clients remained for more extended help. Although mental health problems were extensively present, only just over half were primarily mental health cases. Social problems, particularly emotional and relationship problems were also extensively present. Intervention, with its emphasis on psychosocial methods, reflected this. Having briefly examined the agency as a whole, we may now turn to the analysis of the work of CPNs and social workers.

Chapter 4

Brief Intervention

There are a number of reasons for examining brief intervention separately from more extended intervention. The first may be related to what — in a broad sense — may be called theoretical differences. Brief and extended work represent different philosophies of practice. Advocates of brief work have tended to emphasize the importance of time limitation, engaging the client in the 'here and now' on their immediate problems rather than a deep search for causes involving complex intra psychic therapy (Rappaport, 1970; Reid and Epstein, 1972). Advocates of extended intervention have frequently emphasized just such deep analysis (Yelloly, 1980), while more lengthy intervention may also be associated with the development and sustaining of relationships (Keith-Lucas, 1972). Of course advocates of these approaches often have particular and clear ways of conducting intervention. These were not necessarily being followed specifically by the Centre Workers. Indeed much brief intervention at the Centre would involve only one or two contacts — shorter even than some advocates of brief intervention often consider. However, this theoretical division does highlight different emphases in practice, that different approaches may be made relating to the duration of intervention.

The second reason is more pragmatic: different kinds of cases often require different kinds of approaches, and this may include duration of intervention. Research and practice (Goldberg and Wharburton, 1979; Fisher, Newton and Sainsbury, 1984; Briscoe *et al.*, 1983), have consistently shown that some cases are, by their very nature, chronic and a matter for long term support. On the other hand much briefer work may occur with clients with relatively straightforward problems (e.g. welfare rights queries) or those who require support over a discrete period of change or crisis. The third reason relates to agency function. A significant dimension of the centre's work was its assessment and gatekeeping role, the latter involving referring clients on to appropriate community resources, and which, by its nature, generally involved brief work. This was enshrined in an administrative division between 'brief' and 'caseload' work, which is reflected in this research. This chapter, therefore, will concentrate on the work defined by the agency as brief, comparing intervention undertaken by CPNs, by social workers and

Table 4.1   *Primary Problem of Clients Receiving Brief Intervention*

	Social Work	(expressed as %) CPN	Joint	Total
Mental Health	50	60	50	52
Social/Physical Health	50	40	50	48
p = 0.513[+]				

[+] Chi squared test has been utilised to test for significance throughout the study except where Fisher's exact probability test was appropriate.

jointly, the last involving a combination of two or three of the different occupations of social work, doctor and CPN. Work undertaken by doctors alone is excluded, consistent with the concentration on CPNs and social workers.

Altogether 210 clients fall into this group: 123 (59 per cent) were seen jointly, forty-four (21 per cent) were seen by CPNs forty-two (20 per cent) were seen by social workers. Nearly all brief clients (94 per cent) were seen in under a week, and 89 per cent involved either one or two interviews. The division of labour enables us to examine two essential questions: is joint work in any sense 'superior' to individual work — do clients receive a better service? and are there any differences in the way social workers and CPNs work?

The Client Group

The social characteristics of brief clients did not differ greatly from all referrals, although they appear slightly more disadvantaged. Only 41 per cent of brief clients had the support of a partner compared with 45 per cent of total referrals; 26 per cent were owner-occupiers compared with a third of total referrals, and 53 per cent were in council or owner-occupied — and hence more stable — housing, compared with 64 per cent of total referrals. The unemployed constituted 57 per cent of brief clients compared with 53 per cent of total referrals, while a correspondingly higher proportion (67 per cent) of brief clients received state benefits. There is, therefore, a consistent trend, although none of the differences is significant. This trend occurred consistently across professional groups, which did not differ significantly although social workers, unlike the other groups, saw more females (55 per cent) than males. Social characteristics appear therefore to have had little impact on choice of worker.

Client Problems

Using primary problems to define the client,[1] it is interesting that despite the mental health setting, only slightly over half were mental health problems ('mental health cases'), indicating the importance of social problems in a community setting and perhaps unsurprising in view of the clients' social disadvantages. Only 2 per cent of social or physical health primary problems were ill health, hence the overwhelming majority were social problems. The groups, furthermore, were similar in their distribution of clients: CPNs did identify rather more mental health problems, although differences were not significant. This similarity has a bearing on joint work, which involves greater human resources, and is presumably justified by an accretion of skills or judgment. This raises an issue which should be considered in the following analysis: is there a difference in the service clients receive which justifies the greater resources used? do assessments and interventions vary?

A closer examination of the broad divisions in both the mental health and social primary problem areas ('social problems cases') reveals no significant group differences. The most prevalent problems overall were emotional and relationship (39 per cent) and neurotic/personality disorders (25 per cent), together comprising nearly two thirds of clients, and again occupying that grey area of minor mental illness/severe emotional problems. Psychotic problems were a significant minority (18 per cent) while practical problems, interestingly given the social disadvantage of clients, comprised only 7 per cent of cases. Although not significant there were differences of emphasis. A third of CPN cases were neurotic or personality disordered compared with 21 per cent of social work and 24 per cent of joint cases. Nearly half (48 per cent) of social work cases were emotional or relationship compared with 27 per cent of CPN and two fifths of joint clients.[2] Even examination of detailed problem areas reveals no significant differences and few noticeable variations. Marital problems were dealt with most frequently jointly (12 per cent), compared with under 5 per cent of CPN and social work cases. Another difference was with social relations and isolation problems, comprising 14 per cent of social work and 11 per cent of joint cases but no CPN cases. The greater emphasis on relational problems by social workers reflects a core element of social work practice, and skills in this area have a high profile in social work training. The distribution of marital problems may relate to the nature of the problem: because of the dyadic nature of marital difficulties, two workers, particularly of different sex, may have been considered more appropriate. In the broad area of neurotic problems, their greater prevalence amongst CPNs is consistent with the particular orientation towards mental health in occupational training.

However, these are trends rather than significant differences. Overall, the main impression is one of interchangeability of these groups. To a considerable degree these groups worked with the same range of primary problems. Rather than restrict themselves to particular areas each group adopted a wide role encompassing most areas of work. This provides some evidence for the emergence of the generic 'mental health worker' advocated in particular in some CPN literature (Simmons and Brooker, 1986). This, of course, has major implications for both professional role and training. It becomes possible for two groups to justify their claim to the same 'occupational territory'. The corollary, however, is that individual occupations cannot sustain a claim to exclusive control of practice in particular occupational territory.

Mental Health Problems

For this position to be upheld, however, further analysis of professional role is required. Alongside the primary problem, most clients suffered a number of associated problems. Where mental health problems were identified, they were defined by the workers as either definite or borderline cases, a division used by Brown and Harris (1978) in their study of depressed women (see Appendix 1 in this volume). The frequency with which mental illness was identified was greater than that evident from primary problems: hence the presence of mental illness did not necessarily mean it was considered the primary problem. Again, however, the frequency with which it was identified by the different groups was remarkably similar, ranging between 74 per cent for joint work to 71 per cent for social work (p = 0.950). This was also evident in the distribution of definite and borderline cases. A large majority of each group's clients — 67 per cent of CPN, 60 per cent of social work and 57 per cent of joint cases — were considered only borderline. Taken overall clients seen briefly are perhaps better conceived as suffering acute distress rather more than definite mental illness, which may have contributed to the brevity of intervention.

In terms of broad divisions, between psychotic, neurotic/personality disorder, and alcohol/drug problems, the similarities of each group stands out. Each group identified neurotic problems most frequently — ranging from 37 per cent of joint to 42 per cent of CPN clients — followed by psychotic problems (18 per cent of CPN, 20 per cent of joint and 21 per cent of social work clients), while the rest suffered alcohol or drug abuse. More detailed analysis of individual mental health problems emphasizes still further the similarity of these groups. In no area was there a significant difference between the groups (and many were very similar). Depression was most frequently identified, in a fifth of clients with mental health problems, followed by schizophrenia, alcohol abuse and affective psychosis, all about a tenth of cases.

Social Problems

A changed picture emerges here, with marked differences between different groups becoming apparent. Emotional and relationship problems — markedly the most prevalent — were identified extensively by all three groups

Table 4.2   Broad Social/Health Problem Areas

	(figured expressed as %)			
	Social Work	*CPN*	*Joint*	
Practical	26	56	37	p = 0.016
Emotional/Relationship	81	78	88	p = 0.230
Physical Ill Health	10	25	25	p = 0.094

(table 4.2). However, social workers dealt significantly less with practical problems.[3] The ill health problems reflect occupational role: doctors and CPNs are health professionals, and their training and background are consistent with a greater interest in this area. However, the relatively small proportion of practical problems identified by social workers is a surprise: their training and work skills would be expected to lead to a high profile for this kind of work, rather more than CPNs. Indeed this suggests a lack of emphasis on the practical problems of clients reminiscent of Wootton's classic critique (emphasized also by Howe, 1980) that 'to establish a "good relationship" with the client ... marks a person as a good social worker. *Providing practical help and advice does not*' (Wootton, 1959). CPNs identified them most frequently, social workers least frequently, and joint workers in between. Social workers appear to have adopted a form of 'sub-social casework' counselling role emphasizing emotional and relationship but not practical problems, despite the social disadvantage of clients.

Examination of detailed problem areas bears this out. Social workers most frequently identified emotional and relationship problems: social relationships and isolation (43 per cent), emotional (38 per cent) and marital problems (29 per cent). Amongst CPNs, emotional and relationship problems were also extensively identified — emotional problems in exactly three fifths and social relations and isolation in two fifths of clients — as was the case with joint workers, who identified emotional (62 per cent of cases), social relations and isolation (47 per cent) and marital problems (29 per cent) most frequently. However, they also identified practical problems frequently: financial and housing problems were identified respectively for 33 per cent and 31 per cent of CPN clients, while housing problems were identified for 24 per cent of joint clients.

A further measure of group differences can be made through the concept of 'case complexity'. This is measured in terms of three characteristics: the number of problems, the severity of those problems, and the breadth of the problems. The first represents the number of problems per case suffered by clients. The second relates to the rating made by the workers: they were asked to distinguish between those problems they considered 'severe' and those they did not. The third relates to whether or not problems suffered by different clients were situated in one or more broad areas — practical, emotional and relationship and ill health. When the client had problems situated in more than one broad area they were called 'multi-problem clients'. In terms of broad problem areas nearly two thirds (65 per cent) of CPN and three fifths (57 per cent) of joint clients were multi-problem, but this was the case with only 36 per cent of social work clients (p = 0.06, just below a level of significance). CPN clients averaged 1.58 and joint workers 1.5 problems compared with only 1.16 for social work clients. The picture is similar with detailed problem analysis: CPNs averaged 2.8 and joint workers 2.76 problems per client, compared with only 1.93 per social work client. Interestingly, the position is different for *severe* social and health problems: social workers averaged more of these per case (0.6) than CPNs (0.49), though far fewer than joint workers (1.23). Analysis of case complexity does not therefore present a straightforward group profile. Although clear differences emerge, they are not entirely consistent. Without adopting a rigid formula, however, it appears joint work involved, on the whole, more complex cases, but that while CPNs identified a greater breadth and number of problems than social workers the reverse was the case with severe problems.

Case complexity does appear to provide some justification for joint work. It may indicate greater ability to make an overall assessment, evident through a more complex identification of problems, by bringing together varied skills and perspectives. However, it may also be that joint workers take on cases which appear more complex at referral and their assessment simply reflects this. We can analyze this by examining the referrals. The average (detailed) number of problems identified by referrers was 1.12 for cases allocated to social workers and joint workers and 1.5 for those allocated to CPNs. If we examine the ratio of problems identified by the workers to the number of problems identified by the referrer, we have an indication of the independent problem identification made by the workers (represented by the excess of worker identified problems over referrer identified problems). These ratios were, for joint work 2.35:1, for CPNs 1.86:1, and for social workers only 1.65:1. CPNs therefore did identify a greater number of problems than social workers but the gap between the groups is less in these ratios than when we simply examine the number of problems per case. Most significant though is that joint work did in fact lead to a greater amount of independent problem identification, and hence clear differences emerge in the process of assessment.

Cause

The workers were asked to identify what they considered was the main cause of their client's problems, which was divided up to indicate the broad orientation of the workers. Four main causes were distinguished. The first was 'personal' causes, where responsibility for the problem was attributed to the client. The next two causes go beyond the individual to the social environment. Practical causes involved material factors such as poverty,

Table 4.3   Workers' Perceptions of the Cause of Clients' Problems

| | (expressed as a %) | | | |
	Social Worker	CPN	Joint	Total
Personal	29	38	28	30
Social-practical	12	27	17	18
Social-relational	45	24	40	38
Biological	14	11	15	14
p = 0.323				

financial difficulties, transport problems etc. while relationship causes involved the clients' social network; the unexpected loss of a loved one, the behaviour or attitude of relatives or friends and so on. The final area was biological, where the problems were attributed to biophysiology or the medical condition of the client.[4] This broadly reflects Mitchell's (1974) distinction between psychological, social and biological factors. Although there were variations between different groups, these were far from statistically significant (table 4.3). Indeed, even controlling for primary problem divided between mental health and social problems, these groups are characterized by their similarities rather than differences. More detailed division into broad areas of mental health and social problems likewise revealed no significant differences. The overall emphasis on social causes — consisting of over half the cases — is consistent with the degree of social disadvantage, both material and relational, evident in the client group. It is interesting, however, that relational causes were identified nearly twice as frequently as practical causes, despite the severe material disadvantages of many clients. Indeed personal causes are given a considerably higher profile than social practical causes. Although this evidence is only suggestive, and in view of the particularly wide gap between social, practical and personal causes identified by CPNs and social workers, personal causes may reflect a belief that their situation was a product of the client's own behaviour rather than vice versa. This view is perhaps surprising in social work, which has a long tradition, even in social casework, of considering the social context of behaviour (Hollis, 1972; *cf.* Corrigan and Leonard, 1978; Bailey and Brake, 1975). An interesting difference is the greater emphasis by CPNs compared with social workers on the practical rather than relational element of social environment. This is consistent with the more extensive identification of practical problems by CPNs, and suggests a greater orientation on their part to practical matters than social workers. The slightly greater emphasis by CPNs on personal causes is consistent with the more individualist approach evident in nursing literature, while social workers in particular, but also joint workers, more frequently identified relational causes than CPNs. These, however, were trends and not statistically significant.

Another way of examining social environmental problems is in terms of whether they were sudden, possibly unanticipated events, such as burglary or unexpected marital desertion, or more long term persistent problems like poor housing or income. The social disadvantage of clients, particularly material but also relational might be expected to lead to an emphasis on longer term causes of the clients' problems. This was not the case: social environmental causes were equally divided up between events and difficulties by social workers (19 per cent each) and CPNs (20 per cent each) while joint workers identified more events (23 per cent) than longer term difficulties (16 per cent) as causes. A distinct crisis element appears therefore in workers' perceptions of client referrals. Hence the focus was not simply directed extensively to the individual but also circumstances likely recently to precede the referral: the focus appears limited therefore both contextually and temporally. Of course a background to these events may have been long term difficulties and the events may have acted as the 'final straw' (*cf.* Brown and Harris, 1978). It is possible, for example, to envisage the parent struggling to care for a family on inadequate income reacting very negatively to a robbery or a very heavy bill.

Client Management

Context of Intervention

Client management refers to the different approaches made by workers to intervention with the client: similar to that described by Bartlett (1970) as 'interventive repertoire'. The context for intervention refers to the social context within which client intervention takes place. This may be considered in terms of degree of 'social distance' from the client themselves at which the intervention takes place. In effect this involves examining the social context in which intervention takes place, and is divided up in terms of intervention which focuses on the client alone, the family of the client, their friends or acquaintances, and community professionals or agencies.[5]

This may be usefully represented diagrammatically (see figure 4.1). Intervention for each client was defined in terms of the widest social context in which intervention took place. Hence, if intervention only involved interviews with the client alone, this was how the case was defined. If, however, interviews occurred with the family as well as the client, the context was defined as 'family level'. The intervention context at further social distance from the client subsumed all context closer to the client: hence if intervention involved work with agencies or professionals, this subsumed all other contexts. There were, as with most other aspects of work, no significant differences between the groups in their context of intervention (p = 0.345). Overall 79 per cent of clients were dealt with at the community-agency level, while most of the rest — a further 18 per cent — involved seeing the client alone. However, the CPNs did rather more work with client alone (24 per

Figure 4.1 Context of Intervention

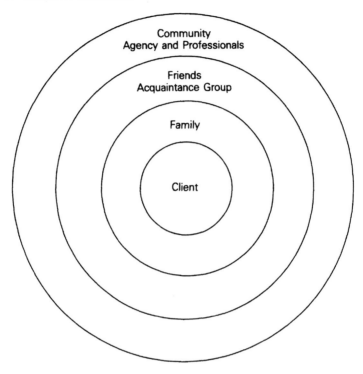

cent of their cases) than either social workers (19 per cent) or joint workers (15 per cent). On the other hand, joint work more frequently involved community-agency work (83 per cent of cases) than social workers (74 per cent) or CPNs (71 per cent).

However, if health agencies and professionals are excluded from the community agency level — hence we concentrate on non-health community agencies and professionals — these differences become significant (table 4.4). Overall the exclusion of health agencies and professionals radically reduces the proportion of clients seen at community-agency level (to 25 per cent) and increases those seen at family level (to 24 per cent) and work involving the client alone (to 49 per cent). Clearly all three groups showed a strong orientation to health agencies and professionals. However, social workers worked with non-health agencies more than joint workers and markedly more than CPNs. At the same time, they were less likely to limit intervention to the client alone, or the family acquaintance and group levels. The greater the influence of social workers on decision making, the greater was the emphasis on non-health agency work; thus it occurred most frequently when social workers were exclusively responsible, less frequently with joint responsibility and least frequently with CPN responsibility. This is not,

Table 4.4   Level of Intervention — Excluding Health Agencies

Level of Intervention	(figures expressed as %) Social Work	CPNs	Joint
Client alone	45	56	48
Family level	17	20	28
Acquaintance-group		7	1
Non-health community-agency	38	18	23

p = 0 038

perhaps, surprising. CPN training and self perception is of a health professional, whereas social work maintains a greater emphasis on the social context. This is interesting because it highlights a disjunction between the identification of practical problems which occurred with greater frequency in the CPN clients, and their preparedness to work with non-health agencies. Frequently such agencies, such as DSS, housing dep tment or even Citizens Advice Bureau, will be of considerable significance in the management of practical problems.

Problems Tackled

Problems tackled by workers give a further indication of the context of intervention. Workers were asked to indicate when they identified social and health problems, whether they tackled these problems, and if these were tackled indirectly. Problems were defined as indirectly tackled when they were worked on without involving the client, such as contacting outside agencies on their behalf or working with others in their social network, without the client's presence. Whether examined in terms of broad problem areas, or detailed social problems, the groups are again noticeable for their similarity. Although, with one exception, social workers tackled identified problems most frequently, the differences were far from significant. Problems tackled indirectly showed a similar pattern. It is noticeable indeed that problems were frequently not tackled at all by all three groups: social workers tackled two thirds or fewer of problems identified in seven out of twelve problem areas as did CPNs and joint workers with eight (out of eleven) and eleven (out of thirteen) problem areas respectively. Fifty per cent or less were tackled by social workers in four, CPNs in six and joint workers in seven problem areas. This limitation is still more marked with indirect work. All twelve areas identified by social workers and eleven out of thirteen identified by joint workers were tackled with a frequency of under 40 per cent. CPNs tackled all problem areas identified with a frequency of less than 33 per cent. This may reflect a combination of the brevity of intervention, and the assessment and gatekeeping role of the centre, by which client problems were

Table 4.5 Roles Adopted by Workers

	(figures expressed as %)			
	Social Work	CPN	Joint	
Assessor	45	58	57	p = 0.381
Drug administrator	—	2	5	p = 0.282
Psychosocial treatment and support agency	31	27	37	p = 0.451
Teacher/counsellor	69	78	68	p = 0.430
Broker/advocate	17	20	25	p = 0.472

assessed, and then were referred on to other agencies. The task, in these cases, would not necessarily be to tackle the problems, but to identify them and then refer to an agency which would tackle them.

Role and Activities

The activities undertaken by workers have been clustered together, using Whittaker's (1974) typology, amended to embrace the activities of the health workers other than social workers at the centre,[6] to indicate the roles adopted by the workers (table 4.5). Again, however, there are no significant differences between the groups, providing further evidence for the inter-changeability of the professionals. The teacher–counsellor role was that most extensively taken by all three groups and may be related to the brevity of intervention. This role, involving in particular the provision of information and advice and discussing future options, may provide necessary initial help before referring clients on to other agencies. Alternatively, when clients are not referred on, this role may provide an immediate 'boost' to the client, clarifying available options to enable them to manage their problems themselves. The limited amount of assessment is surprising in an advice service. This may in part reflect previous acquaintance with the client. Altogether 69 per cent of clients were previously known to the psychiatric services, and many of these may have been known to the worker or their colleagues. In these cases detailed assessment and examination may not have been considered necessary. Some problems, furthermore, may have been considered relatively straightforward and not requiring detailed analysis. The work of psychosocial treatment agent reflected monitoring and emotional support rather than psychodynamic work, less appropriate with brief intervention. The limited broker-advocate role, when considered in relation to fairly extensive contact with outside agencies and professionals indicates that this contact was primarily information giving and referral rather than assertive espousing of the client's case. Drug administration was rare, reflecting the

Table 4.6 Activities Undertaken: Significant Differences

| | (figures expressed as %) | | | |
	Social Work	CPN	Joint	
Section assessment	17	—	18	p = 0.010
Assessment/exploration	27	58	42	p = 0.022
Mobilizing resources	10	18	21	p = 0.024

need for continued supervision not available with brief intervention, and was, of course, not undertaken by social workers.

More detailed activity analysis shows social workers most frequently discussing future options (48 per cent of clients), providing information and advice (45 per cent) and emotional support and ventilation (31 per cent). Assessment and exploration was most frequently performed by CPNs (58 per cent of cases), while information and advice and discussing future options occurred in 56 per cent of cases. Future options were discussed in 53 per cent of joint cases while information and advice and assessment occurred in 45 per cent and 43 per cent of cases respectively. Some significant differences were evident (table 4.6). Given legal requirements, it is not suprising CPNs undertook no section assessments, and the reduced number of other assessments by social workers may be explained by section assessments on other occasions. The limited resource mobilizing by social workers is consistent with the limited identification of practical problems.

The workers were asked to indicate the activity they considered to be most effective. As with most other areas there was no significant difference between the groups. The role considered to be most effective (in between two fifths and a half of cases) was that of teacher counsellor, followed by assessor, effective in just under a quarter of cases.[7] Analysis of individual activities also reveals no significant differences. The most frequently effective activities overall were the provision of information and advice and discussing future options (both 22 per cent of clients). Significant differences were evident in only one activity: assessment and exploration, considered most effective in 22 per cent of CPN cases compared with 10 per cent of joint and 7 per cent of social work cases (p = 0.049).

Cases Referred On

The gatekeeping role of the centre, designed to aid access to a variety of community resources, meant that cases referred on represented an important aspect of its work. These were clients whose needs were assessed and then referred to agencies or professionals considered most appropriate to help them further. Altogether 153 (73 per cent) cases were referred on in this way.

For only a minority of cases, therefore, was brief intervention on its own considered sufficient. This is not surprising in view of the mental health needs and social problems of these clients. However, as with other areas of work, the frequency with which clients were referred on did not vary greatly between groups: 69 per cent of social work, 72 per cent of joint and 78 per cent of CPN clients were referred on. Furthermore, clients were generally referred with a similar frequency to particular agencies. Noticeable differences occurred with 'in patient' referrals comprising 22 per cent of joint and 24 per cent of social work referrals but only 7 per cent of CPN referrals ($p = 0.056$, just below significance) but this may be related to the compulsory admission role of social workers and doctors. A further 16 per cent of CPN referrals but only 4 per cent of joint and no social work referrals went to CPNs ($p = 0.004$). This appears related to professional contact and identity: CPNs showing a greater proclivity to refer on to their own professional colleagues. However, no further significant differences were evident. Thus, both in terms of frequency and destination of referrals, these groups operated similarly as gatekeepers.

Does closer analysis, however, reveal differences? The division of clients by primary problem into mental health and social problem cases again shows no significant differences. Primary problem rather than occupational group provide the key to differences. Nearly all clients with psychotic primary problems — 34 out of 35 — were referred on, compared with only 24 per cent of alcohol/drug and 25 per cent of neurotic — personality disorder cases. In relation to social problem cases nearly two thirds (64 per cent) of emotional and relationship, and two fifths of practical problem cases were referred on.[8] The presence or absence of mental disorder also had an impact on decisions to refer on, though again there was little variation between groups. Clients suffering a mental illness were significantly more likely (77 per cent) than those not (61 per cent) to be referred on ($p = 0.027$). Mentally ill clients were clearly seen as more 'in need'. Nonetheless, a significant minority (23 per cent) did not receive further help either within the centre or from outside agencies and professionals. Only one (out of forty) psychotic client was not referred on, hence the overwhelming majority of those with mental health problems who received only brief help suffered neurotic/personality disorder or drug/alcohol problems. This is interesting because it provides a rough gauge of the seriousness with which different problems were regarded.

The limitation of work with non-psychotic clients with a mental illness to brief intervention may result from various possibilities. Some may have been considered to have sufficient and adequate social supports, which would provide an alternative to formal professional support, particularly where resources were limited. There is extensive evidence to show social support can have a buffering or preventative effect on the onset of mental illness (Henderson, 1984; Mueller, 1980; Frydman, 1981). Alternatively, workers may simply have felt that not all non-psychotic clients required further help

— that their personal resources were sufficiently great, after some initial help, to manage their own problems. It may, furthermore, represent a moral judgment in which the client is somehow 'blamed' for their problems and left to resolve it themselves. Rees (1978) has shown how moral judgments can have a major impact on social work decision making in area teams. This is consistent with causes which emphasize the personal responsibility of clients discussed earlier. One further possibility — that these problems were considered resolved — may be dismissed: workers very rarely considered mental health problems resolved with brief intervention.

The behaviour of the different groups varied little also in relation to social problems. Unlike mental health or primary problems, however, there was no positive relationship between the presence or severity of social problems and decision to refer on. Indeed, although differences are not significant, if any trend existed, it was an *inverse* relationship between the presence of social problems and decisions to refer on. Multi-problem (defined in terms of broad problem areas) clients were less likely to be referred on than others: 83 per cent of clients with no social problems and 73 per cent of clients with one or two problems in broad social problem areas were referred on, compared with 59 per cent of those with problems in three areas.

Two overall conclusions may be made. First the nature of the problem rather than the occupation of the worker is significant in understanding the decision to refer on. Second, mental health problems — particularly psychotic — rather than social problems were positively related to the decision to refer on.

Outcome

The issue of outcome in relation to intervention was very much based on the workers' own perspectives. This is consistent with the overall approach, which has been to examine the work of the different occupations in terms of occupation appropriate meanings, and to emphasize the way the workers themselves construct their practice. The central concern then, was to examine how much change overall, had been achieved and with which problems they perceived most change to have occurred. This was undertaken on a case by case basis, in which workers indicated in relation to the problems they identified how much change they felt had occurred. On the basis of their responses, an 'index of change' was developed in relation to particular problems and a global rating for overall intervention. The index of change was based on an arithmetic formula, which involved giving numerical values to particular outcomes. In relation to the problem categories, the following alternatives were available to the workers, which were subsequently given the accompanying numerical values.

Mental Health Problems		*Social/Physical Health Problems*	
No improvement	0	No help	0
Improved	1	Helped	1
Resolved	2	Solved	2

Measurement of brief intervention emphasized the notion of helpfulness of the worker. This was conceived in terms of helped or not helped: if no help was given a score of 0 was ascribed, if some help was given a score of more than 0 was achieved. Hence the measures only examined positive change. In relation to mental health the notion of 'improvement' was used to indicate where help was given (as was 'helped' for social problems) but, given the brevity of intervention it was more a measure of initial reduction in intensity or number of symptoms. Both 'resolved' for mental illness and solved for social problems were used to indicate where the problem had been reduced to a point where it was no longer considered by the worker to be a problem. In the case of mental illness, it was recognized from early preparation of the project and meetings with practitioners that resolved problems were likely to be rare.

For any particular problem, the formula was:

Sum of score of all cases where the problem was identified ÷ The number of cases where the problem was identified = Index of change

For broad problem areas the formula was extended to an aggregation of all problems in the relevant area. Hence 'practical' social problems included financial, housing, employment and home management. An aggregate score would be attained by adding together the score for all occurrences of the problems and dividing it by the frequency with which these problems occurred. Since negative scores were not possible, the minimum score in any area was 0 and the maximum was 2.

Brief intervention was not, on the whole, seen to be helpful with mental health problems (table 4.7). Overall, and this was the case in particular with CPNs and joint work, they saw themselves as most helpful with neurotic problems. However, given that the maximum possible mark was two, even with neuroses this help was generally rather marginal. While no group saw themselves to be particularly helpful with mental health, it is noticeable that in *no* cases did social workers consider themselves to have helped with mental health problems. Furthermore, while the importance of medication to the treatment of psychosis makes the perceived lack of helpfulness with these problems unsurprising, it is interesting that all three groups considered they gave no help to those with drug or alcohol problems. These may have been regarded as responsive only to longer term work, or it may reflect a view that these problems were self inflicted (hence raising the moral issues of

Table 4.7   Index of Change: Broad Problem Areas

	Social Work	CPN	Joint
Psychotic	0.000	0.000	0.042
Neurotic	0.000	0.263	0.200
Alcohol/drugs	0.000	0.000	0.000
Overall mental health	0.000	0.152	0.110
Practical	0.424	0.080	0.228
Emotional/relationship	0.230	0.283	0.220
Ill health	0.500	0.182	0.097
Overall social/health	0.273	0.273	0.198

deserving and undeserving as discussed earlier) and workers may consequently have been less concerned with helping. More detailed analysis of individual mental health problems merely serves to demonstrate further the low level of perceived help. Social workers felt they had helped with no problems, CPNs with only depression (0.600) and anxiety (0.250) and joint workers with depression (0.160), anxiety (0.625) and schizophrenia (0.091).

The scores for social and health problems indicate that the workers felt more able to help in these areas. Overall they felt most helpful with emotional and relationship problems, but there was considerable variation between different groups. Care should be taken when comparing groups because these are essentially subjective assessments and the criteria used by different groups to make these assessments may vary. Nonetheless, it is interesting that in two out of three areas the social workers scored themselves more highly than the other groups. Although identifying fewer practical or ill health than emotional and relationship problems, social workers considered themselves more helpful with the former. Joint workers considered themselves marginally more helpful with practical than emotional and relationship problems, while CPNs considered themselves most helpful with emotional and relationship problems. These results are interesting when considered alongside the frequency with which these groups dealt with these problems. In particular the high score for change by social workers with practical problems was associated with a low frequency of identifying these problems. However, it is consistent with social workers' greater involvement with the community-agency context of intervention, an appropriate venue for intervention with many practical problems. The helpfulness of other groups was more closely associated with the frequency of identifying problem areas: in particular the high score given to emotional and relationship problems. The evidence suggests that, although they identifed practical problems less frequently than other groups, when involved they frequently considered themselves particularly able to help.

More detailed analysis of social and health problems reveals social workers considered themselves most helpful with housing (0.625), minor physical ill health (0.667), emotional (0.412) and child abuse problems (0.333). CPNs helped, they felt, most with emotional problems (0.333), loss and separation (0.200). Joint workers scored most with emotional (0.316), child care (0.333) and housing problems (0.267).

Conclusion

Examination of brief intervention reveals a complex relationship between occupation, role and behaviour. Our analytical framework provided three alternatives in relation to professional behaviour. First, occupational training and expectations — the process of socialization and accruing professional knowledge — may lead to clear differences between occupations. Second, however, the knowledge and skills base may be sufficiently uncertain, and require extensive use of judgment such that differences would be blurred as individuals respond to uncertain situations where clear processes of intervention are not obviously available. Third, contact between occupations — particularly where knowledge and skills have an element of uncertainty — may lead to 'seepage' of knowledge and approaches between different occupations resulting, with sufficiently close contact, in narrowing of occupational differences.

Such differences, which might reflect clearly demarked 'professional worlds' did occur. Some were in directions predictable from our analytical framework. In particular work at the non-health community-agency level was carried out by social workers significantly more than CPNs. This is consistent with more detailed examination by social work of intervention in the social environment. Likewise, although the differences were noticeable rather than significant, the greater emphasis by CPNs and joint workers on physical ill health is consistent with greater health orientation than is evident in social work. Other differences, however, do not appear consistent with our framework. CPNs identified significantly more practical problems than social workers, a surprising finding in view of the clearer emphasis in social work of examination of the social environment, and the context of intervention undertaken by each group. Case complexity, with CPNs and social workers, did not point in one direction. CPNs identified on average more problems than social workers, and also more multi-problem clients (defined in terms of number of broad areas). However, they identified fewer severe problems than social workers.

The main impression, despite these differences, is the degree of similarity between these groups. They showed this in a number of key areas. There was a similar distribution of primary and mental health problems, and although differences were evident in social problems in relation to practical difficulties, all three groups identified emotional and relationship problems most frequently. Likewise, although differences were evident in a small number of activities, the roles adopted by the groups differed very little.

Finally, the cause attributed by different groups to clients' problems varied little. Very frequently, there was a high degree of crossover between the groups: hence the same problems were identified most frequently by each group. Each group, furthermore, carried out a whole variety of activities. This tends to point to the importance either of 'seepage' or the uncertainty of the knowledge or skills base. The possibility of 'seepage' was clearly available. The centre had operated for a number of years, and there was a high degree of interprofessional contact at a number of levels. They occupied the same building which encouraged interaction and relationship building; problems relating to specific cases, and indeed broad issues of practice, were frequently discussed in some detail; and perhaps most important joint intervention was extensively undertaken. This, in particular, would entail joint involvement in all aspects of intervention, facilitating joint decision making and management of cases. Such processes would encourage the exchange of ideas in terms of defining the client and the process of intervention. These may encourage the development of a similar range of alternative constructions of situations. Such seepage would be facilitated by a knowledge base, whose status is uncertain. The difficulty of 'fit' between knowledge base and practice situations creates a 'space' of uncertainty in relation to particular cases filled by practice experience and judgment. Individuals attempting to manage these situations with limited knowledge guidance would have room for interpretation. Where individuals from two occupations have close contact, they may develop similar ways of constructing situations, resembling each other both in their interpretation of, and characteristic responses to, situations.

Two further related issues arise. Joint work might, by incorporating different professional perspectives, provide a wider assessment and intervention repertoire. Certainly, the complexity of joint worked cases was greater than individual occupations, and more problems were independently assessed. However, in other respects joint work differed little from social work or CPN intervention. An alternative possibility is the advent of the generic mental health professional, in which social workers and CPNs are effectively interchangeable. A good deal of evidence for this has been produced, providing support for the claims of the newer CPN profession to areas of work formerly the territory of social workers. However, these conclusions relate to brief intervention. The very brevity of the intervention may act to supress differences which, with longer intervention, would become apparent. The next chapter will address this issue.

Notes

1   Workers were asked to identify which of the range of mental health and social problems which a client suffered, they considered to be their primary problem: this provided a helpful way of defining clients, in terms of workers' perceptions.

2 Mental health problems were divided into three broad categories: psychotic, neurotic and alcohol/drug abuse (see Appendix 1). Social problems were divided into three broad categories: practical, emotional/relationship, physical ill health (Fitzgerald, 1978). When mentioned in the text 'broad' categories refer to these, while detailed categories refer to the detailed classification of mental health and social problems (see Appendix 2).

3 A difference is considered significant if there was less than 1 in 20 likelihood that it was the result of chance, i.e. $p < 0.05$.

4 The constituent elements of each cause on the research form were

Personal: Behaviour/attitude of the client;

Social-practical: Sudden practical event; persistent material/practical problems; persistent ill health/disability problems in client/relatives;

Social-relational: Sudden relationship event; behaviour attitude of relatives/acquaintances/friends; combined behaviour of client/relatives/acquaintances;

Biological: Psychophysiological; failure to take prescribed medication.

Persistent ill health or disability refers to ill health or disability in the client or relative which had lasted for some time (a number of months or possibly years). It was described as social-practical because it was currently or likely in the future to involve impaired functioning of the individual. Furthermore, health is a social as well as biological concept (Freidson, 1970). In these respects they differed from organic or biochemical bodily disorder underlying a mental disorder, which was defined as psychophysiological.

5 In relation to context of intervention the categories on the research form were:

Client alone: Interviews with the client alone;

Family level: Interviews with spouse or family; interviews with client plus spouse or family;

Acquaintance-group: Interviews with friends or acquaintances; interviews with client plus friends or acquaintances; group work;

Community-agency: contacts with outside agencies and professionals.

6 Whittaker divided these roles up into treatment and support agent, teacher-counsellor, broker and advocate. To these were added assessor, because of the important assessment function, and drug administrator, since there is an aspect of the CPN role. The activity categories for each role were as follows: assessor — section assessment, other assessment and information gathering; drug administrator — one activity; psychosocial treatment and support agent — psychodynamic work, ventilation and emotional support, monitoring; teacher/counsellor — education in social skills, providing information and advice, discussing future options; broker/advocate — mobilizing resources, advocacy on behalf of client.

7 Teacher-counsellor: social work 50 per cent, CPN 46 per cent, joint 42 per cent of cases;

  Assessor: social work 21 per cent, CPN 24per cent, joint 24per cent of cases.

8 Ninety-eight per cent of primary social problem clients were either practical or emotional and relationship cases.

Chapter 5

Extended Intervention

Both practical and theoretical reasons have been put forward to explain the separate analysis of brief and extended intervention. The most pervasive, however, relates to the agency itself: the division reflects the way the agency defined cases, and hence the reality of the workers' own experience of intervention. In addition to brief intervention, cases were allocated to the caseload of individual workers, either 'short term' or on a more long term basis. Short term cases were those generally expected to involve three or four visits following the initial assessment. However, boundaries were blurred as some short term cases developed into long term work, and those designated long term at times involved relatively few interviews. Some cases designated short term were not classified long term when additional interviews occurred because of the extra administrative work involved. Hence, caseload cases have been analyzed as a total group. Analysis of brief intervention created an intriguing picture: that, to a considerable degree, there was little difference in the role and behaviour of separate occupations (or combinations of occupations). The issue of occupational difference was not finally resolved, however, because of the brevity of the intervention. Further light may be thrown on the issue through more extended intervention. While the data on brief intervention were based on cases referred during a four month period, data on extended intervention involved cases referred over a one year period (see Appendix 1).

The Client Group

Noticeably more clients (eighty-four) were allocated to social workers than CPNs (fifty-nine). There were no significant differences between CPNs and social workers in the age or sex of their clients. There were, however, more females (57 per cent of clients) than those receiving brief intervention. Almost all clients (97 per cent) were aged from 20 to 64, reflecting the age range appropriate to agency function. Differences did exist in other areas

Table 5.1   Mental Health Cases: Broad Problem Areas

	(expressed as %) Social Workers	CPNs
Neurotic/personality disorder	44	79
Psychotic	38	3
Drug/alcohol	12	18
Uncertain	6	—
p = 0.004		

indicating two trends. First, social work clients tended to be more disadvantaged than CPN clients. Fewer social work clients (48 per cent) were in potentially supportive relationships (married or cohabiting) than CPN clients (68 per cent, p = 0.026). Second, slightly more social work (35 per cent) than CPN clients (27 per cent) were unemployed, while of those in work, 76 per cent of social work and 67 per cent of CPN clients were below social class 2.

Client Problems

Primary Problems

CPNs defined significantly more of their clients' primary problems as mental health — mental health cases — than social workers. Social/health problems were primary in 81 per cent of social work clients[1] compared with 44 per cent of CPN clients (social problem cases). Conversely, 56 per cent of CPN and 19 per cent of social work clients' primary problems were defined as mental health (p < 0.0001). The net result of this was that overall ninety-four clients (66 per cent of total) were considered to be social problem cases and only forty-nine to be mental health cases. A major role difference — or way of defining the client which implied a role difference — is apparent, in which mental health was given a higher profile in defining CPN clients, while social workers gave an overwhelmingly higher profile to social problems. The more even distribution of CPN clients between mental health cases and social problem cases — although CPNs nonetheless more frequently gave priority to mental health — indicates less exclusivity in their approach. The number of social problem cases shows that their involvement with these problems was perceived to be a legitimate aspect of their role. It reflects a concern with social aspects of psychiatry which has been strongly advocated in the CPN literature as a major aspect of working in the community (Carr, Butterworth and Hodges, 1980; Simmons and Brooker, 1986).

More detailed analysis reveals further interesting and significant differences. In relation to mental health cases (table 5.1) CPNs overwhelmingly concentrated on neurotic clients, and the majority of other mental health cases had alcohol or drug abuse problems, which were invariably not psychotic in nature. Within this neurotic group, anxiety had a major profile: it was the primary problem for nineteen CPN clients, accounting for nearly three fifths of mental health cases. To a considerable degree this relates to CPN's skills based interests: behavioural work, relaxation and 'anxiety management' techniques are important tools in CPN intervention with anxiety (Thyer, 1987) as is the use of cognitive methods with depression (Alloy, 1988). These represent techniques applicable to specific problems, with clear methods as procedures. Hence, to deal with anxiety through relaxation tapes is not to confront other problems in the clients' social circumstances that they may suffer. There is a hint here of compartmentalized skills specific to particular problems. This may lead to some inflexibility — that whatever other problems are present, the one with which the profession has relatively narrow skills (in a spectrum of client problems) will be that focused on. This would reflect an emphasis on skills but not on theory which would place those skills in the context of professional role which links those skills in a repertoire which may be used with a client (Bartlett, 1970). This issue may be examined further later in relation to activities, role and context of intervention.

The CPN predilection for choosing neurotic cases is not evident in social workers, who were allocated a wider range of cases, and were considerably more likely when involved with mental health cases to take on psychotic problems. These are often defined as the major mental illnesses and are often as much a matter — in psychosocial as well as medical treatment — of maintenance rather than resolution (Leff and Vaughn, 1984). The limited involvement with psychotic problems by CPNs may in certain respects represent what David Howe (1986) has termed 'ditching the dirty work'. 'Dirty work' according to Hughes (1958) is work which is in some sense distasteful, and as a consequence less valued than other work. It may be physically disgusting, such as waste removal, morally dubious, such as associating with stigmatized groups such as prostitutes or simply carrying out tasks which others would prefer not to do. Hughes argues further that any occupational group wishing to enhance its status will choose its work carefully, in particular avoiding work which may be assigned the designation of 'dirty'. Howe (1986) argues that 'people' work may be dirty in two respects: either what is being done *or* with whom it is being done. Cleaning bedpans or the consequences of incontinence are examples of work activities which are 'dirty'. Working with highly stigmatized groups, such as criminals, may also be 'dirty'. In this case working with psychotic people may represent the dirty end of work with the mentally ill (who are as a whole a group suffering from stigma).

Indeed the process of concentrating on 'clean' work has occurred in nursing, where higher status jobs — particularly the managerial side of nursing — have become particularly valued, and basic physical care has been relegated to nursing auxiliaries (Carpenter, 1977). The selection of clients on

Table 5.2   Social Problem Cases: Broad Problem Areas

	(figures expressed as % of cases)	
	Social Workers	*CPNs*
Practical	2	11
Emotional/relationship	96	85
Health	2	4
p = 0.071		

the basis of what they can do for the practitioner or profession has been called 'creaming' (McKinlay, 1975). The selection of clients at the 'clean' end of the spectrum of work is a process which is designed to help occupational mobility. In the case of the CPNs this may be enhanced in various ways. The first is by moving to higher status work: in this case it would involve emphasis on the less stigmatizing neurotic rather than pyschotic problems. Second, this involves moving away from areas more likely to be subordinate to medicine. The psychoses generally involve some kind of drug maintenance and have overall medical supervision. Neuroses can involve less or no use of medication: for example anxiety can be dealt with by relaxation or behavioural techniques. Finally, the emphasis with psychotic problems is to a considerable degree maintenance. Work with neurotic problems may offer more scope for positive change. The fact that the agency was not under overall medical supervision, will, to a considerable degree, have given the workers greater opportunity to choose their clientele and hence professional role. In this case the CPNs seem to have chosen the more status enhancing and rewarding cases.

The greater range of primary mental health problems undertaken by social workers is also evident in relation to individual psychiatric problems: social workers identified eight different types of mental health primary problems compared with only five by CPNs. This, it will be remembered, was the case in relation to a significantly smaller number of mental health primary problems identified by social workers. Indeed, the greater emphasis on anxiety in particular by CPNs was highly significant (p = 0.0004). There were, therefore, major differences between CPNs and social workers.

The differences between social workers and CPNs in the distribution of social primary problems — though less marked than mental health primary problems — were nonetheless noticeable and just below a significance level (table 5.2). Social workers displayed an almost exclusive concentration on emotional and relationship problems, and although the differences are small the greater CPN interest in practical problems reflects a trend evident in brief intervention, and is perhaps similarly surprising. Overall, the primary problem in over four fifths of both social work and CPN clients were defined in the area of neurotic-personality disorder, emotional and relationship problems. This confirms a trend in brief intervention and indicates that this 'space' of severe emotional distress–minor mental illness was not simply that characteristic overall of the agency, but in all aspects of work. If the client group as a whole is examined (rather than dividing it up into mental health and social problem clients), and detailed problem areas are analyzed, the largest number of social work primary problems were clients with emotional (24 per cent), loss or separation (29 per cent), and marital problems (14 per cent). All these are indicative of personal crises or the disruption of social and emotional supports. Amongst CPN clients anxiety, comprising just under a third of cases (32 per cent) was the most significant primary problem. Other groups, all constituting between 10 and 12 per cent of the total, were those with marital, loss or separation, emotional, depression, alcohol and drug problems. Although anxiety stands out, other CPN primary client problems also emphasized emotional difficulties or social support disruption.

Mental Health State

Mental health problems could be present even where workers defined the primary problem as non-psychiatric. A client, for example, might be depressed, but their primary problem identified as housing or child care. Hence it is no surprise that mental health problems were identified with greater frequency than they were defined as primary. Nonetheless, the distribution of mental health problems between social workers and CPNs presents a similar trend to that evident in primary problem. Exactly half the social work clients had a mental health problem, compared with over four fifths (81 per cent) of CPN clients, a significantly greater proportion (p = 0.0003). Hence, despite the title of the agency, there was, as with brief intervention, a far from exclusive concentration on mental health problems, and this was particularly evident amongst social workers. Indeed, the attribution of primary problems by the workers indicates that, even when a mental health problem was present, it was not automatically accorded primacy. This is important when we try to understand the construction or meaning these professions place on their work, a matter which will be dealt with in more detail later.

The pattern changes somewhat in relation to the distribution of definite and borderline cases in clients with a mental health problem. While nearly three fifths (57 per cent) of social work clients with a mental health problem suffered a definite disorder, the corresponding figure for CPN clients was 29 per cent. Where social workers identified mental health problems, therefore, they were rated, on the whole, as more severe. Two possibilities present themselves. This may, first, reflect a genuinely greater severity in the mental health problems managed by social workers. Alternatively, when mental health problems were present, social workers may have been more likely than CPNs to define them as 'definite' (they would have had a lower threshold than CPNs). However, both occupations were based in mental health settings and had extensive experience of different 'levels' of mental health problems. Furthermore, the high degree of contact between the two occupations, particularly evident in joint work, but also in sharing the same base, would be expected to create a greater degree of unanimity than might otherwise be the case. The distribution of mental health problems with brief intervention assessments is very similar as between the three groups. Finally, social workers were less likely to identify mental health problems and when identified were less likely to regard them as primary. This does not suggest an occupation whose thresholds, in relation to mental health, were lower than CPNs. It appears likely, therefore, that these differences reflect a greater frequency of definite cases among clients of social workers with mental health problems.

Where mental health problems were present, social workers most frequently identified depression (44 per cent of cases) and anxiety (28 per cent). CPNs likewise identified anxiety and depression most frequently, although rather more anxiety (47 per cent) than depression (32 per cent of cases) was identified. This confirms the emphasis on neurotic difficulties evident in the analysis of primary problem. On the evidence both of primary problems and mental health problems, social workers to a great degree consider — even as specialist mental health workers — mental health to be an aspect of social problems, the management of which represents the core of their training. Indeed, it is perfectly possible to interpret mental health in 'social' terms. Brown and Harris (1978) in their study of depressed women found this to be the case amongst their subjects. I have argued elsewhere, furthermore, that social workers are concerned with mental health primarily as a social rather than health problem (Sheppard, 1990). Mental illness is a state which contravenes norms or standards which are broadly valued. Social workers' involvement derives from a broad social concern with mental illness, as a result of which social workers are empowered to take part in the management of these problems. This is highlighted in terms of their position as approved social workers, where they are directly empowered by statute to act as applicant in relation to compulsory admissions, as well as carrying out other duties. The emphasis on social problem definition is, therefore, consistent with a broad social problem orientation in social work.

Social Problems

There were marked differences also in the realm of social problems. This may be examined first in terms of case complexity. Social workers tended to take on more complex cases in relation to social problems than CPNs. The average number of social problems per case identified by social workers was 4.3 compared with only 3.4 by CPNs. Social workers also identified more severe problems, averaging 2.7 per case compared with only 1.1 per case identified by CPNs. The relative 'gap' between social workers and CPNs (measured in terms of ratio of social work to CPN problems) widened with

Table 5.3 *Social Problems: Broad Areas*

| | (figures expressed as %) | | |
	Social Work	*CPN*	
Practical	56	63	p = 0.525
Emotional/relationship	98	90	p = 0.104
Ill health	23	25	p = 0.851

severe problems. This reflects the tendency, evident in relation to mental health, for social workers to have a higher proportion of mental health problems which were definite disorders and never more severe. However, this trend is not evident in relation to multi-problem clients. Broad problem areas may be used to identify clusters of problems residing in broadly similar areas — practical, emotional and relationship, and physical ill health. Where a client had problems in more than one broad area they were defined as multi-problem clients. The differences betweeen the two occupations in the number of multi-problem clients was small: thus 45 per cent of social work and 47 per cent of CPN clients had problems in two areas while 16 per cent of social work and 17 per cent of CPN clients had problems in three areas. Overall, then, although social workers identified a higher average number of problems per case, the main difference was in greater severity of both mental health and social problems identified by social workers.

The similarity between social workers and CPNs in multi-problem clients is reflected in the types of problem identified. It is, unlike mental health, the similarity of, rather than difference between, the occupations which is marked. Both placed great emphasis on emotional and relationship problems, although practical problems also had a high profile in the client group. Examination of detailed problem categories reveals that those most frequently identified by social workers were emotional (92 per cent), social relations and isolation (62 per cent), loss or separation (60 per cent) and marital (58 per cent). The CPNs identified similar problems although less frequently: emotional (70 per cent), marital (46 per cent) and social relations and isolation (41 per cent). This is, of course, consistent with broad problem areas. However, it also serves to confirm the impression evident from the social and demographic data: that these people were, to a considerable degree, lacking in social support or suffering disruption to their social network. The figures for marital problems are particularly interesting: even those who did have the support of a partner were frequently subject to problems in their relationship with them. There were significant differences: although social workers identified child abuse in 11 per cent of their clients, no CPN clients had this problem (p = 0.025), not surprising in view of the responsibilities of these professions. Interestingly, however, social workers identified significantly more problems than CPNs in a number of emotional and relationship areas. Thus, they identified significantly more emotional (p = .001) and

Table 5.4   Cause of Problems

	(figures expressed as %) Social Work	CPN
Personal	25	20
Social relationship	59	54
Social practical	8	17
Biological	8	9
p = 0.4586		

social relations or isolation problems (p = 0.020), as well as problems of loss or separation, identified in only 25 per cent of CPN clients (p = 0.0001). This serves to emphasize still further the ubiquity of these problems in the social work client group.

Severe social problems present a different picture. In relation to broad problem areas, social workers identified practical problems in 26 per cent and CPNs in 22 per cent of their cases; ill health was identified in 11 per cent of social work and 9 per cent of CPN cases. Neither difference was significant. However, emotional and relationship problems showed a highly significant difference: 93 per cent of social work clients, but only 49 per cent of CPN clients suffered these problems (p < 0.0001). Almost all social work clients, therefore, had at least one severe emotional or relationship problem. A more detailed breakdown shows highly significant differences in relation to marital, loss or separation, social relations or isolation, and emotional problems.[2] Social work cases, it seems, presented considerably greater difficulty in the realm of emotional and relationship problems.

Cause

Although there were considerable differences in the types of problems identified, the attribution of cause by CPNs and social workers showed very small variations (table 5.4). As with brief intervention, social relationships were given a high profile. However, differences *between* various casues are exaggerated by comparison with brief intervention. Personal causes, though still important, were identified with considerably less frequency than social relationships, which dominated as a cause. The gap, in the realm of social environment, between practical and relationship causes is very wide, and particularly so in the case of social workers. Interestingly there is little difference between CPNs and social workers in their ascription of biological causes, indicating that social workers were able to 'take on' domains beyond the purely psychological. There is further evidence here of a surprisingly small emphasis placed on practical causes, noted in relation to brief

Table 5.5   *Context of Intervention (Excluding health agencies)*

	(figures expressed as %)	
	Social Work	CPN
Client alone	17	51
Family level	15	22
Acquaintance-group	17	5
Community-agency	51	22
p < 0.0001		

intervention. Indeed CPNs identified rather more practical causes than social workers.

Role and Context

Context of Intervention

There were major differences also in the nature of intervention undertaken by CPNs and social workers. The variation between the two occupations at the family level of intervention was small: 6 per cent of social work and 5 per cent of CPN cases were managed at this level. The differences at community-agency level were also small, involving 70 per cent of social work and 76 per cent of CPN clients. However, rather more CPN cases (19 per cent) than social work cases (11 per cent) involved working with the client alone, and while 13 per cent of social work clients were managed at the acquaintance-group level, this was the case with no CPN clients. These differences were significant (p = 0.023) but they were not straightforward. Our framework suggested that the more individualist CPN approach would manifest itself in the tendency to work with the client alone and eschew the use of outside agencies and professionals in the community. Social workers, on the other hand, would be expected to have greater involvement with outside agencies and community supports. In fact, while the CPNs did limit their intervention to a greater extent to the client alone, they nonetheless involved the family and outside agencies to as great an extent as the social workers. Indeed the emphasis amongst social workers on the acquaintance-group level reflects to some degree the interest in group work. On the basis of this evidence, the CPNs were both more likely to work with individuals alone yet equally likely to involve outside agencies and professionals.

The exclusion of health agencies and professionals changes the picture markedly, (table 5.5). The overall trend shows that the greater the 'social distance' from the client at which the intervention took place, the greater the excess of frequency of social work involvement over CPN involvement.

Thus a considerably greater proportion of social work than CPN clients were subject to intervention at community-agency level. Intervention with the client alone was practically a mirror image of that at community-agency level: showing a marked excess of CPN over social work intervention. These differences emphasize, first, by comparison with social workers, the individualist orientation of CPNs. Second, they indicate that, by comparison with brief intervention, the social workers were more prepared to respond to clients' needs by working with outside agencies. This appears to suggests greater interest in working at a resource level with practical problems.

However, analysis of contacts with key outside agencies indicates limits to the work undertaken by social workers with more material and financial problems. Contact with the DSS or housing department occurred in only 10 per cent of social work cases, perhaps surprising in view of client social disadvantage. This can be examined further in relation to clients who were unemployed, or employed but on state benefit. These were the more deprived clients, who might be expected to have greater contact with the DSS or housing department. Although contacts with this group were more frequent than those not in this situation (six out of nine clients for whom these contacts were made were unemployed or on state benefit), this was not a significant increase in frequency ($p = 0.156$). Equally pertinent was the proportion of cases where clients were unemployed or on state benefit where contact was *not* made. In over four fifths of such cases (82 per cent) such contact was not made. These figures indicate limitations on the otherwise noticeable involvement by social workers with community agencies and professionals, which occurred primarily with agencies other than DSS or housing department. Although, therefore, social workers were, by comparison with brief intervention, more involved at the community-agency level, Wootton's (1959) criticism, noted in relation to brief intervention is relevant also to long term work.

The separation of health from other agencies and professionals helps to explain the level of community-agency involvement by CPNs. It appears the most significant factor in relation to involvement with outside agencies was their health orientation, which seems at times to have overridden their more individualist tendencies. This may indeed involve — in part at least — the residue of a former subordination to the medical profession from which the CPNs have been struggling to free themselves. This would be the case if they were referring to doctors in circumstances where they might have made independent decisions. Indeed, CPNs were remarkable for their degree of medical consultation. In 73 per cent of cases CPNs made contact with a GP or consultant psychiatrist. Thus medical liaison was involved in *nearly all* cases where community-agency intervention took place. Although this does not mean they were always seeking advice or guidance — it may often have involved information giving — this suggests they placed great importance on contacts with doctors in case management. Social workers by contrast showed more independence (or less interest in communication). They had

Table 5.6   Proportion of Problems Tackled Indirectly: Broad Problem Areas

	Social Workers	CPNs	
Practical	34	16	p = 0.111
Emotional/relationship	42	11	p = 0.0002
Ill health	32	27	p = 1.000

contacts with these doctors in only 38 per cent of their cases, significantly fewer than CPNs. Of course interprofessional communication is generally highly valued (DHSS, 1978). The degree of concentration by CPNs on contact with doctors by comparison with contacts with other agencies indicates this did not arise because of general ability to communicate well with others. It may well be that, although seeking greater independence than in the past, they have not managed to break the umbilical cord with medicine.

The number of contacts with outside agencies and professionals emphasizes further social workers' greater community involvement. Social workers averaged 5.6 contacts per case compared with 2.8 by CPNs. When health agencies and professionals are excluded the difference is more marked: 2.8 averaged by social workers and 0.4 by CPNs. CPN contacts with non-health agencies were, therefore, very rare indeed. Intervention by social workers, which will be discussed later, did tend to last longer, and this may have some relevance for the number of outside contacts.

Problems Tackled

Problems tackled, particularly those tackled indirectly, give a further indication of the context of intervention. Most problems were tackled by workers. In seven of the eleven problem areas identified by social workers — housing, marital, loss or separation, social relations or isolation, emotional, criminal behaviour and child care — over four fifths of client problems were tackled. In all other areas — except major physical ill health where only two fifths were tackled — a minimum of two thirds were tackled. The picture was similar with CPNs. In all but two problem areas — home management and criminal behaviour — a minimum of three quarters of identified problems were tackled. Consistent with evidence on intervention context, social workers manifested a greater tendency than CPNs to tackle problems indirectly, that is where the client was not present (table 5.6). In the realm of ill health the two occupations were notable for their similarity. This was not the case with emotional and relationship problems, where social workers managed significantly more problems indirectly and practical problems where they were noticeably, though not significantly more frequently indirectly involved. The greater amount of indirect work by social workers with practical

Table 5.7   Professional Role

	(figures expressed as % of total client group)		
	Social Workers	CPNs	
Assessor	93	70	p = 0.0006
Drug administrator	—	12	p = 0.0045
Psychosocial treatment and support agent	94	85	p = 0.1195
Teacher/counsellor	92	88	p = 0.6791
Broker of services/advocate	38	3	p < 0.0001

problems is consistent with social workers' greater involvement with non-health agencies and professionals. The limited indirect work by CPNs with emotional and relationship problems is surprising: by their very nature relationship problems involve others in the clients' social network. It suggests that a significant aspect of this work — that with others concerned with the relationship problems — was not undertaken. Their work here appears somewhat truncated. More detailed analysis of individual areas shows social workers consistently to have tackled problems indirectly more frequently than CPNs: in eleven out of thirteen problems social workers exceeded CPNs. However, this difference was significant in only two areas: housing and emotional problems.[3] The difference was just below significance with child care and social relations or isolation.

Professional Role

Consistent with the analysis so far, social workers and CPNs manifested significant differences in professional role (table 5.7). The extent to which the teacher–counsellor role was taken varied little between CPNs and social workers, but in other roles there were marked and significant differences. The exclusivity of drug administration to CPNs is not surprising, and reflects their responsibilities. With the exception of advocate and service broker, social workers adopted other roles very widely indeed. While CPNs also adopted the role of assessor in a large majority of cases, it was nonetheless significantly less frequently than social workers. Both occupations adopted this role more frequently than when undertaking brief intervention. It is perhaps surprising CPNs did not assess more extensively: where this did not occur, it necessarily meant a greater reliance on referral information or previous knowledge of the client. However, this lack of assessment was not related to previous knowledge on the part of the psychiatric services — and hence CPNs — of the client: there was little difference in the frequency of assessment by CPNs between new referrals (71 per cent) and those already known (67 per cent). This, then, indicates a preparedness by CPNs in some cases to accept others' definitions of the client, while social workers' greater predilection for assessment suggests a greater degree of independent judgment.

The other significant role difference was as advocate or service broker. The very restricted performance of CPNs of this role further emphasizes their limited work in the community agency context. This suggests that those contacts they made were limited to the transmission and receipt of information. However, social work performance of this role was more restricted than other roles. This indicates the extent to which social work concerns were directed towards achieving change or development in the individual themselves. Taken together with the emphasis on emotional, relationship and neurotic problems, this underlines the degree to which they were involved in personal growth. A more detailed analysis of activities undertaken, rather than broad roles, shows social workers averaging 5.7 activities per case compared with a CPN average of 3.7. The activities most frequently performed by social workers were assessment (93 per cent of cases), ventilation and emotional support (89 per cent), discussing future options (88 per cent) and psychodynamic work (61 per cent). CPNs most frequently undertook the discussion of future options (83 per cent of cases), ventilation and emotional support (73 per cent), assessment (68 per cent) and information and advice (61 per cent). Social workers undertook activities more frequently than CPNs in eight out of ten areas, and significantly more frequently in four areas.[4]

The concentration by CPNs on individuals, their emphasis in particular on anxiety management, and the considerably smaller repertoire of roles and activities undertaken in cases provides strong evidence of a narrower range to the work of CPNs. In effect they were choosing cases in specific areas, and carrying out more limited tasks in a narrower range of contexts than social workers. This is consistent with the emphasis on a more rigid use of skills, and a narrower range of applicable skills suggested earlier. The claims made by CPNs, outlined in Chapter 2, to a very broad biopsychosocial domain are not matched by an ability to work in contexts beyond the individual (the social aspect of the trio of domains) or undertake roles applicable to those contexts. This may well arise because of an overemphasis on particular skills and a poverty of theory development, which would help place those skills appropriately within occupational role.

Most Effective Activity

The perception of most effective activity — the activity which the workers considered most effective in facilitating positive change, maintaining the client, or reducing possible deterioration — did not differ greatly between social workers and CPNs. Both considered their role as psychosocial treatment and support agent most effective in most cases: 69 per cent of social work and 63 per cent of CPN clients. Assessment was considered most effective with a similarly small proportion of clients: 5 per cent of clients. Interestingly, CPNs considered drug administrator to be the most effective role in none of their cases. This may be because of the types of problems clients had, which CPNs may have considered more responsive to alternative methods, or because they saw drug treatment to be generally less effective. An interesting possibility is the distancing of CPNs from one of their traditional roles; part of their attempt to free themselves from medical control. In this context the small number of psychotic cases, where biochemical treatment frequently takes a high profile, and the small proportion of clients who actually received drugs provides further suggestive evidence. Differences did occur in other roles but they were not significant. CPNs considered the teacher-counsellor role to be most effective in 31 per cent of cases compared with 18 per cent of social work cases (p = 0.117), and social workers believed that broker/advocate role was most effective in 8 per cent of their cases compared with 2 per cent of CPN cases. In the teacher counsellor role the biggest differences appear in the more didactic elements: information and advice and education in social skills were considered most effective in 14 per cent of CPN but only 5 per cent of social work cases. There was, it appears, slightly greater value placed by CPNs on aspects of work which involved instructing the client.

Interviews and Intervention

There were major differences between CPNs and social workers, both in the number of interviews undertaken and the length of intervention. Social workers averaged 4.4 months per client compared with the CPN average of only 2.9 months. When the duration of intervention is graduated the difference is significant. Nearly a fifth (19 per cent) of CPN clients were seen for under a month compared with 8 per cent of social work clients while 23 per cent of social work clients but only 3 per cent of CPN clients were seen for *over* six months (p = 0.013). A similar picture emerges in relation to interviews with clients and others in their social network: social workers averaged 13.1 and CPNs 6.5 interviews per client. When the number of interviews is graduated, work with over two fifths (41 per cent) of CPN clients compared with only 12 per cent of social work clients involved four or less interviews. However, in nearly half (49 per cent) the social work cases but only 24 per cent of CPN cases more than eight interviews were involved (p < 0.0001). Furthermore, even though they saw clients for longer periods, the *intensity* of intervention by social workers, measured by the average number of interviews per month, was greater than that of CPNs (3.0 compared with 2.2 interviews per month). Overall, then, a client and those in their social network could expect to see lot more of their social worker than CPN. The differences in length of intervention may have related in part to circumstances of case closure. Some clients 'dropped out' of intervention without prior warning: 8 per cent of social work and 24 per cent of CPN clients. The numbers are not, however, sufficient to explain the differences and indeed raise questions about the client–CPN relationship. Some clients were still being seen at the end of the research. The data, however, showing this to be the case with 25 per cent of social work but only 12 per cent of CPN clients further reinforces evidence of social workers greater commitment to longer term work.

Was this variation the result of dealing with different kinds of problems? In most primary problem areas the number of clients seen by one or other profession was relatively small. However, a considerable proportion of both CPN and social work clients' primary problems were emotional and relationship and it is possible to compare them. The trend is generally similar to that for all referrals, although less marked. Work with over two fifths of CPN clients (41 per cent) compared with only 14 per cent of social work clients involved four or less interviews, while only social work cases (14 per cent) involved twenty or more interviews (p = 0.020). Social workers remained involved for longer, although the differences were less marked and did not reach statistical significance. Similar proportions of CPN (59 per cent) and social work (56 per cent) clients were seen for three months or less. However, while exactly a fifth of social work clients were seen for seven months or more this was the case with no CPN clients (p = 0.098).[5] Two conclusions are suggested by this analysis. First, social workers tend to carry out more interviews and intervene for a greater length of time than CPNs. However, when comparison is made when the two professions are working with more similar clients, the differences are not quite so clearcut. This indicates that differences may be more exaggerated when comparing the total client groups of the two professions by differences in the nature of the client groups. Variations between CPNs and social workers, therefore, appear to result both from genuine differences in approach to intervention, and the different types of problems with which they were concerned.

Do these variations in length and number of interviews reflect different philosophies of intervention? Clearly social workers felt their clients needed more intervention than CPNs, but did the nature of intervention vary? It may have been the result of a greater emphasis on the need for support and maintenance of the client or perhaps a more dynamic problem solving approach, with the social worker even, at times, acting as intrapsychic change agent. The evidence is not entirely clear, partly because social workers tended overall to undertake more activities than CPNs: hence it is not simply a matter of CPNs emphasizing certain activities and vice versa. It is certainly the case that social workers emphasized their supportive role; 89 per cent of their clients received emotional support (and ventilation help), compared with a large, but significantly smaller, proportion (73 per cent) of CPN clients (p = 0.020). However, both psychodynamic work, occurring with 61 per cent of clients, and discussing future options, undertaken with 88 per cent of clients were major areas of social work practice. Discussing future options, occurring with 83 per cent of cases, was also an important element of CPN practice. However, psychodynamic work was carried out by CPNs with only one quarter of their clients — markedly fewer than social workers (p = 0.0001). It appears therefore, that differences between social workers and CPNs do not simply reflect different client needs, but different philosophies of practice. The greater length of social work intervention is accompanied by two elements of the tradition for extended intervention. The supportive role indicates workers who acted in a form of long term supportive 'friendship', which to a considerable degree could be related to chronic problems. However, another aspect — the psychodynamic work — appears more closely related to the psychoanalytic tradition in social work, with its emphasis on the resolution of deep seated problems through longer term problem solving work. Indeed, while of course this work may reflect two different approaches made to different cases, it is quite possible for both to be part of the overall problem solving approach, where the emotional support, which might itself have some kind of cathartic effect, provides a foil to the psychodynamic work. Altogether seventy-six of the eighty-four social work cases involved emotional support or psychodynamic work. Nearly two thirds of these clients (66 per cent) received *both* emotional support and psychodynamic work, while nearly a third (33 per cent) received emotional support but no psychodynamic work. Interestingly, this diverges significantly from the forty-seven CPN cases involving emotional support or psychodynamic work. Only 24 per cent involved both activities and 68 per cent only emotional support (p < 0.0001). There is therefore a clear difference between CPNs and social workers. Also, however, these social workers with their greater emphasis on dynamic problem solving differed from the area team workers of the Fisher *et al.* (1984) study, who tended to provide long term support and friendship.

Outcome

The index of change used to examine extended intervention differs in certain respects from brief intervention. The index was designed to measure improvements or deterioration in relation to identified problems, from the beginning to the end of intervention. Hence, workers were asked from their perspective to indicate the direction of change. The measures therefore, were of improvement–deterioration rather than helped–not helped. The following categories were used with associated scores.

Table 5.8   *Index of Change: Broad Areas*

	Social Worker	CPN
Neurotic/personality disorder	0.615	1.077
Psychotic	0.091	0.333
Alcohol/drug abuse	0.000	0.714
Overall mental health	0.415	0.980
Practical	0.452	0.622
Emotional/relationship	0.731	0.972
Ill health	0.158	0.467
Overall social problem	0.659	0.903

Mental Health		*Social Problem*	
Resolved	+2	Marked improvement	+2
Improved	+1	Mild improvement	+1
No change	0	No change	0
Deterioration	−1	Mild deterioration	−1
		Marked deterioration	−2

In relation to mental health, problems were considered resolved where the symptoms were reduced in number and severity to be considered no longer present. It will be noticed also that it is skewed by the inclusion of the 'resolved' category allowing for higher measures of positive than negative change. Both occupations, of course, however, were able to use the same range of measures. The index was worked out using the same formula as that for brief intervention.

The CPNs consistently gave clients a higher rating of positive change than social workers, both in terms of overall change and in relation to broad problem areas (table 5.8). When the overall index of mental health is graduated into cases where the score was above or below nought the difference between the two professions is significant. While 42 per cent of social work cases where a psychiatric disorder was identified scored over nought, this was the case with 78 per cent of CPN clients (p = 0.001). Both social workers and CPNs considered positive change occurred with neurotic-personality disorder problems. However, while social workers considered positive change marginal elsewhere, CPNs on average considered positive change greater with alcohol and drug problems than psychotic problems. This perception of positive change is related more in the CPNs' case to the type of case most frequently allocated than social workers. Social workers, therefore, appear to have been more prepared to accept cases where they considered their help more marginal. More detailed analysis shows social workers to score most highly with depression (0.688) and anxiety (0.600) and least well with mania and alcohol abuse (both 0.000).[6] CPNs scored most highly with anxiety (1.174) and depression (1.000) which formed the great majority of their mental health cases. Other areas are difficult to comment on because numbers were small, although the four alcohol abuse cases averaged 0.500 and the three drug abuse cases, 1.000. In individual as well as overall measures, CPNs therefore tended to identify greater positive change.

Graduating the index of change for social problems also reveals a significantly lower score for social workers: a score of above 0.5 was achieved with 76 per cent of CPN clients compared with 55 per cent of of social work clients (p = 0.017). Both CPNs and social workers identified greatest positive change with emotional and relationship problems, followed by practical and then ill health problems. The CPNs' perception of positive change with practical problems is interesting. Much of their work did not involve roles or contexts obviously related to such work. They acted as advocate or broker of services very rarely, contact with non-health agencies occurred in a minority of cases, and practical problems were tackled less frequently than by social workers. Nonetheless, their index mark is higher than social workers. The basis for this, therefore, is that maybe their greater involvement, by comparison with resource mobilizing, advocacy and indirect work, in giving information and advice and discussing future options. Both of these latter activities may have involved practical issues (such as welfare or employment rights). If so, however, the balance between facilitative advice and direct contact with agencies is perhaps surprising. Up to date information or detailed advice is often best obtained from relevant agencies (e.g. social security agencies or the operation of housing law in a particular area). This is particularly the case in relation to the precise situation or particular problem of the client (e.g. their position on a housing priority list). Low contact with outside agencies would hinder the gathering of such information.

More detailed analysis shows social workers considered most positive change occurred with emotional (1.00), child care (0.76) and social relations or isolation (0.63) problems, and scores lowest with major physical illness (−0.20), criminal behaviour (0.00) and financial problems (0.31). CPNs scored highest with emotional problems (1.14), loss or separation (1.07) and home management problems (1.00) and least with major (0.00) and minor (0.50) physical illness.

The overall results do provoke questions about the reasons for the more positive views on the part of CPNs about change in their clients when compared with social workers. One possibility is that it reflects the severity of problems: social workers identified more of these than CPNs. If so, both groups would be assessing situations similarly, but the index of change would reflect in the outcome of cases the tenacity and intractability of the problems dealt with by the social workers. However, this is not confirmed by the index of change for severe problems, the overall score of which was 0.71 for social workers and for CPNs 1.08. Likewise, while 73 per cent of CPN severe problems were above 0.5, the corresponding figure for social work was 54 per cent. Another possibility is that the differences in scores for change related to genuinely different outcomes: CPNs were actually able to create more positive change than social workers. However, the professionals, and CPNs in particular, are not the only arbiters of this. The views of clients, which may be compared with those of professionals, will be considered later.

A further possibility is that the actual judgments were made differently. This might occur by adopting different criteria to judge change — they would actually look at different factors to judge performance — or by CPNs showing a lower 'threshold' in measuring change. In the latter case a smaller positive change on the client's part would be required by CPNs than social workers to rate improvement to be mild or marked. This is particularly interesting if true (and we shall have further relevant evidence on this from the client), for it suggests the social workers and CPNs operated from different perspectives. This might be expected of course, given differences in occupational culture, training and discourse. However, there was a very close relationship between CPNs and social workers: they were based in the same setting and joint work and discussion were extensively carried out. Taken in the context, in particular of other differences, this suggests that the background training and beliefs derived from work experience left the two professions, if not impervious to changes of view, then at least highly resistant to change derived from contact with other professions. This is not the only indicator of such resistance; clients were defined or chosen differently, while the roles they took and contexts within which they worked also showed marked differences.

Conclusion

The major differences identified in relation to extended intervention indicate that social workers and CPNs took on entirely different roles. Indeed the style of intervention adopted suggests, far from these occupations being interchangeable in terms of community mental health work, that the service to clients would vary greatly according to which profession was allocated the case. The differences confirm, to a considerable degree, expectations arising from the examination of occupational socialization and discourse. Social workers defined their clients primarily in terms of social problems, whereas mental health case definitions received a higher profile amongst CPNs. Social workers, according to the main indicators — role, context and indirect work — operated in a wider community context than CPNs. Social workers acted as advocate or resource mobilizers, worked with outside agencies and professionals, and tackled more practical and emotional and relationship problems indirectly to a far greater extent than CPNs. Indeed, in terms of active use of community resources and agencies, CPN work appears to have been negligible. Where outside agencies were involved CPNs had a particularly strong health orientation although this was noticeable also in the case of social workers. Indeed where agencies and professionals were involved CPNs appeared to have shown a very strong reliance on contact with doctors. The social work task, furthermore, seems to have been more complex. Social workers identified significantly more severe problems, and had significantly more severe multi-problem clients. Social workers undertook more activities per client — they actually 'did more' in client management. Indeed there was a generally narrower range to CPNs' work: they had a narrower range of problems, smaller repertoire of roles, and undertook fewer activities. The number of interviews and duration of intervention undertaken by social workers were greater than CPNs. Indeed, not only was intervention on the whole longer, the *intensity* of intervention was greater by social workers.

Despite this, CPNs associated themselves with greater positive change in their clients than social workers. This is particularly interesting for it suggests an optimistic view of outcome. Such an optimistic view might leave them less inclined critically to assess or evaluate their work, on the basis that it was on the whole successful (alternatively social workers, with a less optimistic view, and perhaps more demanding of themselves, may be more self critical). Social workers, furthermore, were more prepared to accept cases which, on the evidence of the index of change, they were less likely to be helpful.

Overall, therefore, the similarities identified with brief intervention appear very much related to the brevity of intervention. This may be because its brevity did not allow workers to demonstrate a wider range of skills or approaches — there simply was not enough time. Alternatively the range of skills required for brief intervention may have been narrower, and fitted comfortably into the approaches of both CPNs and social workers. However, and this is important for professional image, this may indicate that others may perceive the CPN and social work roles to be interchangeable while this is not, in fact, so. Outside professionals would have a relatively limited contact with CPNs and social workers, and its brevity may have the effect of making the work of these two occupations appear similar.

There were, of course, some similarities. The frequency with which different causes were identified did not vary significantly, as was the case with broad social problem areas. However, the two occupations to a considerable degree adopted different philosophies of practice. Hence social workers undertook more long term work which emphasized emotional support and psychodynamic work, consistent with a psychoanalytically influenced tradition in social work. Indeed the range of social work practice, in view of the, to some degree, limited orientation towards practical areas and the degree of material disadvantage among the clients may be more limited than expected, perhaps emphasizing a more psychotherapeutic counselling role (even though they had a wider community role than CPNs). However, there is some suggestion that CPNs were more rigid in their approaches, arising from narrower skills rather than theory emphasis. Hence their narrower range of work was matched by fewer activities and limited repertoire of roles. Theoretical approaches which had a broader community orientation and that linked skills which could be used in different community contexts may have widened the approaches they made. This conclusion is very much in line with evidence from the literature on nursing models.

Examination of extended intervention, therefore, suggests that although they do have a role of their own, CPNs are not well positioned to take over the traditional social work role. This is particularly interesting because of the close collaboration in much of their work between CPNs and social workers. It may be that this collaboration has sufficient impact to affect practice over a relatively short period of time. However, individual responsibility over a longer period of time clearly demonstrates differences. If 'seepage' of ideas did occur they did not have sufficient impact to make differences insignificant. Although these results are striking, we have not yet heard from the clients. Before doing this, we must examine the foundations for interpersonal skills — the relations with clients — in the respective professional literature, which provide a framework for examining clients' views. Indeed, the knowledge foundations of social work in particular, often considered to be vulnerable to the 'shifting sands' (Stevenson, 1971) of social science, appear considerably firmer than some theoreticians might have us believe.

Notes

1 Physical ill health was the primary problem in only one social work and one CPN client.
2 Marital — social work 46 per cent, CPN 15 per cent, (p = 0.0002); Loss or Separation — social work 48 per cent, CPN 14 per cent, (p < 0.0001); Social Relations and Isolation — social work 35 per cent, CPN 10 per cent, (p = 0.002); Emotional — social work 68 per cent, CPN 31 per cent, (p < 0.0001).
3 Housing: social workers 59 per cent, CPNs 13 per cent (p = 0.047); Emotional: social workers 21 per cent, CPNs 5 per cent (p = 0.043).
4 Assessment: social workers 93 per cent, CPNs 68 per cent, (p = 0.0005); Psychodynamic: social workers 61 per cent, CPNs 25 per cent, (p = 0.0001); Ventilating/emotional support: social workers 89 per cent, CPNs 73 per cent (p = 0.02); Advocacy: social workers 33 per cent, CPNs 0 per cent, (p < 0.0001).
5 Other emotional/relationship intervention lengths:
 Under a month: social work 9 per cent, CPN 14 per cent; 1–3 months: social work 47 per cent, CPN 45 per cent; 4–6 months: social work 24 per cent, CPN 41 per cent.
6 The score of 1.000 for dementia is not mentioned because it involved only one client.

Chapter 6

Practice Foundations:
Interpersonal Relations

This book has emphasized that, if we are to examine and compare social workers and CPNs, this must be undertaken in terms meaningful to these professions. The examination of clients' views, although carried out through field research with clients, may follow the same process. This allows us to judge and compare these professions in terms of approaches and standards which they set themselves. These expectations are presented in social work and nursing literature largely in terms of interpersonal relations.

There are well recognized differences between social work theory approaches, and some debate over the relationship between social science and social work. However, there is a high degree of consensus about the importance of the ability to make and maintain relationships as the basis for all forms of social work, even those which emphasize technical skills (Reid, 1978). Indeed, they form a large proportion of a recent book entitled *The Foundations of Social Work Practice* (Anderson, 1988). Haines (1981) comments.

> Skills in relationships permeate the whole of social work practice, and are one of the essential attributes of the social worker. (p. 130)

This applies regardless of setting, theory or method (case/group/ community work). Perlman (1957) calls the relationship a 'condition in which two persons with some common interest between them. . . . interact with feeling.' Likewise, Kadushin (1983, p. 48) calls it 'the emotional interaction between people'. Unlike friendship, however, the social work relationship is not an end in itself. It is, first, characterized by *purpose*: Pippin (1980, p. 36) maintains it 'is always purposeful' and its purpose is enabling the client. This is presented in general terms by Keith-Lucas (1972) who likewise sees it as facilitative and 'has as its primary purpose the enabling of . . . active and willing choice'. Others see it in more precise terms: it is 'a means by which more specified assistance may be given' (Collins and Collins, 1981) a view reflected elsewhere in an individual context:

The purpose of a professional relationship is to enable a person to work on some specified problem. (Perlman, 1979, p. 64).

The relationship, then, is the foundation for practice, which allows diverse forms of intervention to take place. Additional to its utilitarian dimension, however, relationships have an ethical dimension: according to Ragg (1977, p. 11) it 'should be seen as the seedbed of the primary ethical values of social work'.

Purpose, however, is only one element of the relationship. It should, first, be *open*. Pippin (1980) suggests

> there should be no hidden agenda, no goals towards which the worker is striving which have not been both recognized and agreed with the client. (p. 36)

This involves, as far as possible, that the client takes (some) responsibility, and hence exercises choice. Where not immediately possible, the worker should try to facilitate clients taking responsibility (Moffett, 1968, p. 37). The relationship is also *professional*. As a result, in certain respects the worker appears as an authority figure. He is, first, an official and this should be recognized and incorporated into the relationship, but nonetheless he should attempt to be approachable and receptive (Haines, 1981, p. 139). One dimension of their authority derives from social workers' 'social control' function (Day, 1981) for example when assessing for the compulsory admission of a mentally disordered patient (Sheppard, 1990). However, even when control is absent, authority is derived from knowledge and skills. Perlman (1979) writes

> The essential condition that gives anyone the right to be designated 'professional' ... is that he has some expertise about the problem and about how it may best be dealt with. (p. 72)

The relationship may, however, be seen as *one or two way*. Both Haines (1981) and Keith-Lucas (1972) consider it mutual. 'There are things' states Keith-Lucas 'which the helped person brings to it, and things which are brought by the helping person'. However, Perlman (1979, p. 275) contrasts the 'ordinary life relationship' with the professional relationship, where personal gratification is irrelevant to purpose: 'the client is the one to be served ... *his* needs are to be met not ours'. Likewise, Bessel (1971, p. 23) states social workers offer 'a one way therapeutic relationship' and Pippin (1980, p. 52) argues 'it is for the client and not the worker'. This may not be a contradiction: rather, different aspects of the relationship may be emphasized. On one hand, helping, like 'ordinary' relationships, requires a two way affective dimension, on the other the worker should nonetheless be clear that it is primarily for the client. Finally, the relationship is not static but a *process*:

like Haines (1981) and Siporin (1975), Compton and Galloway (1979) comment that relationships have

> motion and direction and emergent characteristics. It grows, develops and changes and when the purpose has been achieved it comes to an end.

Nurses are also interested in relationships but manifest less coherence and display greater fragmentation. Different orientations to the client are discussed in nursing literature around three interrelated areas: communication, the nursing process and inter-personal and social skills. The fragmentation arises largely within the context of nursing's attempt to escape the control or influence of medicine. Nurse authors make much of conflicting demands of the more medically oriented versus interpersonal approaches. Bottorff and D'Cruz (1984) distinguish a patient centred from an interpersonal approach. The patient centred approach, they say, is 'in reality an illness/disease based approach' activities are directed by the disease/disability of the patient and 'the interpersonal-social-relational domain languished through neglect'. Yuen (1984) relates this to two different approaches: an 'authoritarian' approach, where patients are 'managed according to a system of hospital regulations' and conformity is expected and a 'therapeutic community' approach requiring 'the maximum of freedom' and a 'spontaneous sharing and expression of real feeling'. However, nursing has, according to many authors, been dominated by more medical models: this means that emphasis has been placed upon learning about disease and treatment. Likewise Crowe (1982) suggests that nursing is traditionally

> almost exclusively care oriented following the medical model of disease, with an emphasis on institutional care concerned with acute episodes of illness.

Psychiatric nursing appears no different from other aspects of nursing. Reynolds (1985) states that 'United Kingdom [psychiatric] nurses have poor role clarity'. Furthermore, their practice frequently reflects the model identified by Crowe. Cormack (1976) suggested psychiatric nurses' main purpose for involvement with clients was to gather clinical data relating to their symptoms. Indeed, many of the profession themselves appear to have regarded psychiatric nursing primarily as common sense. Nurses frequently have no easily identifiable perspective to guide them (Altschul, 1972). Sladden (1979, p. 30), drawing on research, comments on the theoretical or ideological rootlessness of psychiatric nurses. Psychiatric nurses appear to be differentiated in respect to their attitudes to treatment methods, not by their own clearly held approach, but according to the predominant approach of the hospital in which they work. Sladden comments that community based nurses *may* have more discretion (though this is not helped by theoretical rootlessness).

The literature on nursing as a whole tends to subordinate counselling — which provides a focus for relationship work — to a relatively peripheral activity (although this literature will be examined later). Its fragmentation is emphasized by the notion of 'nurses as counsellors' rather than viewing counselling as an automatic element of nursing, as relationships are for social work. Dartington *et al.* (1977) declare that counselling skills are not intended

> to prepare nurses to be counsellors but to enhance their counselling skills within the professional role.

Barry (1984) in a book *specifically about* psychosocial nursing states that merely

> with a *basic* [my italics] knowledge of counselling theory and a warm, caring approach to patients you are in an excellent position to help your patients.

Indeed Stewart (1975) describes nurses as professionals who are taught that they should *not* show their feelings, and to make decisions *for* rather than *with* their patients. This is called 'professional distancing'. Flaskerind *et al.* (1979) identify strategies nurses use actually to avoid closeness with patients such as concentration on impersonal aspects of care, not being involved in direct care, or seeking promotion. It is, thinks Barry (1984, p. 142) the 'constant exposure to illness and death' which leads to these forms of defence mechanism.

There have been greater aspirations to use interpersonal process in psychiatric nursing. Pepleau suggested as long ago as 1962 that they should be specialists in interpersonal techniques and counselling should be part of nurse skills, taught in basic training (Pepleau, 1962). However, the basic psychiatric nursing literature is marked by the *absence* of such techniques (e.g. Burr and Andrews, 1981; Altschul, 1978; Trick and Obcorskas, 1980; Ritter, 1989). Airdoos (1985) comments that:

> acquisition of interpersonal and communication skills are inadequately addressed in undergraduate and diploma [psychiatric] nursing programmes.

It is noticeable that psychiatric nursing literature is not more advanced than general nursing literature in the analysis of interpersonal processes. Psychiatric nurses — if they use nurse authors — are therefore reliant on general nursing literature for guidance in this area. It is unsurprising that 'disease' models exercise such influence.

The fragmented and ambivalent approach of nursing to interpersonal approaches, then, contrasts markedly with social work's impressively consistent emphasis on the relationship as fundamental to practice. Nonetheless, there exists relevant literature in both disciplines. There is a range of elements identified, which may broadly be divided into two. First some may appear as attributes of the person: empathy, genuineness, authenticity and so on (relationship qualities). The second may appear as skills or knowledge based: adviser — expert, therapeutic and so on (expert skills). This does not mean that the first group does not involve skills — indeed they may be developed through appropriate training — rather that they draw on qualities which may appear 'naturally' in some people.

Communications

Although communication skills of the sort discussed here fall into the second group, they provide a useful preamble to the discussion of other elements in both groups. We are concerned to *communicate* relationship qualities such as empathy and genuineness as much as expert skills like advice. Both social work and interpersonal nursing literature emphasize communication. For social work, Haines (1981) comments that

> it is clearly of the utmost importance that effective communication
> be established between social worker and client (p. 170)

Nurse authors think likewise (a nurse in Bridge and Mcleod–Clark, 1986, p. vi) 'communication is not an optional extra . . . but a central feature in the role of the nurse' while Speight (1986, p. 86) considers it 'vital for psychiatric patients' well being'.

Both groups recognize its problematic nature derived from the difficulty in understanding and transmitting meaning. Porritt (1984, p. 13), a nurse, comments 'we cannot be sure the same word has the same meaning for two individuals'. Compton and Galloway (1979, p. 104), social workers, consider it (*cf.* Satir, 1964) 'an interactional process which gives, receives and *checks out* [my italics] meanings'. The main division, reflected in both literatures is between verbal and non-verbal communication (Compton and Galloway, 1979; Porritt, 1984; Kagan *et al.*, 1986; Smith and Bass, 1982). Verbal communication is made through speech, while non-verbal is (Smith and Bass, 1982, p. 83) 'all that is perceived by the senses except the words that are spoken, heard or read'. It can involve, for instance, touch, body movement, smell and paralanguage (speech intonation, etc.). It is the *combination* of verbal and non-verbal messages through which communication occurs, sometimes called symbols (Smith and Bass, 1982). Transmitting and receiving these depend on, according to some (Kagan *et al.*, 1986, p. 52) our 'schemata' — our expectations, our stereotypes and implicit personality theories.

Social work writers have distinguished a number of *levels* of communication. Hollis (1972, p. 6) and Compton and Galloway (1979, p. 205) distinguish overt from covert (corresponding to verbal and non-verbal) messages. Satir (1964, chapter 8) distinguishes denotative messages — the literal content of symbols (usually words) from meta-communication, which is messages about messages (voice inflection, gesture, manner of speaking, etc.). They also discuss the *process* of communication. A number (Kadushin, 1983, p. 44; Compton and Galloway, 1978, p. 205; Brown, 1973) identify various stages: encoding, transmitting and receiving/decoding the messages. Similar dimensions are identified by nurse authors (Smith and Bass, 1982; French, 1983) together with the requirements of schemata, and levels of communication, the process makes communication subject to possible distortion and confusion. This increases in likelihood with people from different cultures (Hollis, 1972, p. 26). French (1983), a nurse, emphasizes the importance of heightened awareness of meaning and possible distortion by nurses, while Middleman and Goldberg (1974, pp. 125–7) identify social work skills to combat confusion: checking out inferences and assumptions, giving feedback, amplifying subtle messages and toning down strong messages. Overall then, both nurse and social work writers display awareness of the subtleties, possible distortions, but great importance of communication and hence communication skills.

Relationship Qualities

Acceptance

Acceptance, and its associated value of being non-judgmental, is extensively examined in social work. It involves 'respect and concern' (Kadushin, 1983, p. 59) and 'an uncompromising belief in the innate worth of the individual human being' (Bessell, 1971, p. 37). It is essential not simply that the worker should have these beliefs, but that the client actually *experiences* himself being respected by the worker (Pippin, 1980, p. 27). Acceptance, however, does not give the client licence for anything. Perlman (1979) considers this leaves the relationship non blaming and non censorious — 'I accept you but not your acts'. Both Bessell (1971, p. 37) and Timms (1964, p. 21) likewise distinguish the client from his behaviour

> it is possible to accept the person even though the case worker may have to make clear ... that certain behaviour is in his view bad.

Perlman (1979) suggests we do not, therefore, display *unconditional* positive regard: there is an expectation by the worker that change will occur. Acceptance, however, requires *humility*. Ferrard and Hunnybun (1964, p. 49) emphasize 'a spirit of humility, induced by a breadth of understanding of human nature and its frailties'. Keith-Lucas (1972) considers it possible because we accept our own fallibilities — that we could have done what the other did if circumstances had differed. Indeed, it may go beyond simple refusal to judge, but actively to seek to understand can be a prerequisite to acceptance (Compton and Galloway, 1979, p. 172). A final element is the commitment implied by acceptance: that although the client may behave in ways disapproved of, the relationship will continue as far as the worker is concerned (Moffett, 1968).

Nurse authors likewise emphasize not judging. French (1983) stresses

consciously attempting to suspend personal value judgments, opinions, attitudes and feelings about the issues raised, and concentrate on accepting the client's values, feelings and opinions (p. 174).

Barry (1984) agrees and suggests the nurse should accept the patient 'as he [sic] is', and Pepleau (1988, p. 29) spells out the implications: in addition to accepting him/her as he is, the nurse should treat the patient as an emotionally able stranger and relate to him/her as such until evidence shows otherwise. Nurse, (1975, p. 38) identifies three elements: nurses must remain true to their values while accepting the patient's right to follow his/her conscience, they must display tolerance of themselves and others and must be non-judgmental so the patient feels free to express his/her real feelings. To be accepting is, at base, to be friendly (Nurse, 1975, p. 58)

the nurse who responds unconditionally ... is a friendly person who encourages the patient 'to expand his first remarks'.

Empathy, Listening, Individualizing

Empathy, listening and individualizing are a closely related cluster of qualities. Empathy is perhaps the most widely discussed element in social work and nursing literature on relationships. Turning first to social work, Haines (1981, p. 152) suggests it is *imaginatively understanding* others: 'the power to feel imaginatively the experience of the other person ... to "get on the same wavelength" as them'. The social worker attempts to 'put themselves in another's shoes'. However, this should not overwhelm them. Biestek (1957, p. 50) calls it controlled emotional involvement, and Compton and Galloway (1979, p. 175) suggest it should occur without losing personal perspective rather using understanding to help others. Perlman (1979, p. 58) identifies a continual movement between merging with the client and regaining an objective stance. We recognize that we are a separate person, and this is necessary to maintain a sense of proportion. There is a clear *intuitive* dimension. Jordan (1979, p. 20) considers 'it requires the exercise of all her [the worker's] intuitive and imaginative capacities' to go beyond the detail of the message. It also has a more *cognitive* element. It involves 'building up our knowledge' (Collins and Collins, 1981, p. 8) and

> methods of reasoning . . . to make an objective analysis . . . [and] the theoretical knowledge [to obtain] . . . a mental representation of the other. (Compton and Galloway, 1979, p. 176)

Through this we gain an understanding of the client's definitions and perspectives: but it must be *accurate* and it must be *conveyed*. It is 'the accurate assessment of another person's definition of the situation . . . conveying that understanding in a genuine manner' (Epstein, 1985, p. 16). England (1986, p. 23) analogizes it to a journey with the client, so the worker knows 'the sights and experiences which the traveller must encounter'.

Listening is a closely associated practice element. Indeed, it would appear a prerequisite to any degree of accurate empathy. Although non-verbal cues may be used, the ability to listen significantly facilitates understanding of the client and the meaning for him of his circumstances. Listening, however, is not a passive activity. Haines (1981, p. 172) emphasizes social work involvement, and the active seeking for 'information': 'a listener who is able to respond actively and appropriately to the messages he receives'. Compton and Galloway (1979) consider likewise

> it is not a passive 'hearing'. It is an active search for the meaning in and and an active understanding of, the client's communication. (p. 168)

It is this active striving for meaning which links it to empathy, the attempt to understand. It is 'listen and know what I mean' (England, 1986, p. 23). Listening, though, has a further positive element: actually encouraging the client to express himself. It involves (Bessell, 1971, p. 19) 'listening hard, not only to the words which the client is using, but also the overtones of what he is saying' together with 'encouraging the client to formulate and express his worries'.

Individualization is also closely associated with empathy: for to empathize is to do so with an individual who has *unique* qualities. Biestek (1957, p. 25) classically defines it:

> individualization is the recognition and understanding of each client's unique qualities . . . based on the right to be treated not just as a human being, but as *this* human being with his personal differences.

Similar definitions are found elsewhere: 'the worker responds to the client as a unique individual' (Kadushin, 1983, p. 57); 'to see the person as a unique human being with distinctive feelings, thoughts and experiences' (Compton and Galloway, 1979, p. 172); 'his uniqueness as an agent' (Ragg,

1977, p. 57). Timms (1964, p. 57) considers individualization possesses two central characteristics: like others it involves a recognition of uniqueness, but also one of *value* — 'a valuation of an individual's potential accomplishments'. Ragg (1977, p. 58) identifies three ways in which it occurs in practice: in the present through the current worker-client relationship; in description of the past through which the client presents their biography; and discussing future actions contributing to his/her personal identity. Overall, Moffett (1968, p. 29) suggests 'treatment should be geared to individual needs ... the caseworker should proceed at the pace of the client'. Above all, individualization means being free from projecting stereotypes on to people.

Interpersonal approaches to nursing also discuss empathy. Kalisch (1971) considers it 'the ability to perceive accurately the feelings of another person and to communicate this understanding to him'. Stewart (1983, p. 45) distinguishes various elements to understanding: it is 'the capacity for participating in a vicarious experience of another's feelings, volitions ... or ideas'. Speight (1986, p. 87) considers it to be an absolutely essential element of interpersonal communication. Like social workers, nurse authors recognize it goes beyond simply what another person says: it is the ability to perceive accurately 'the internal frame of reference' of the other (Tschudin, 1987, p. 33) and involves 'the latent meaning of what has been said' (French, 1983, p. 186). It is necessary, though, to retain some separateness: it is the quality of objectivity Stewart (1985, p. 26) thinks which distinguishes empathy from sympathy. For Ward and Bishop (1988, p. 36) it means, overall 'seeing things through the other person's eyes': it involves, first, responding to the words and reflecting them, and second, picking out the unspoken feelings behind what is said (Tschudin, 1987, p. 33).

Individualization is not a concept discussed extensively in nursing, although an individual's uniqueness is recognized, through, for example, their personality, character, motivation and experience (Stewart, 1985, p. 45). Listening, though, receives greater consideration. At one level, nurse authors examine it in a more basic manner than social work. Pepleau (1988, p. 109) considers it as a 'sounding board' against which the patient can ventilate his feelings. Bridge and Mcleod-Clark (1986, p. 92) likewise consider it 'listening without commenting or questioning'. However, Marks-Maran (1988, p. 40) suggests it is 'much more than social listening' and, like others, uses the term 'attending', through which the nurse gives the patient all her available attention. It goes beyond linguistic communication (French, 1983, p. 170)

> attending is concerned with the verbal and non-verbal cues by the counsellor in response to the verbal and non-verbal initiative taken by the ... patient.

Furthermore, it is active: nurses should not just 'sit passively', but actively let the patient know they are being attended to, heard and understood. Such attending, though, is not straightforward: it is not simply notic-ing verbal and non-verbal cues, but involves *interpreting* these in the total context of the client's situation (Smith and Bass, 1982, p. 174). Overall, Stewart (1983, p. 40) identifies three key elements to listening: awareness of verbal and non-verbal communication; understanding what is said; and awareness of clients' meanings. Irving (1978, p. 33) calls this last 'listening with the third ear': 'picking up the underlying meaning of the message ... and not relying on the obvious or superficial meaning'. She thinks this is the key to skilful listening.

Authenticity — Genuineness — Openness

A further cluster of related concepts discussed in social work are authenticity, genuineness and openness. Kadushin (1983, p. 65) distinguishes between authenticity and the related concept of genuineness. Authenticity requires the worker 'be real and human in the interview. It implies ... spontaneity, the willingness ... to share ... one's own feelings and reactions'. Genuineness on the other hand 'means that there is a striving towards congruence between the worker's feelings and his behaviour'. Authenticity, then, means retaining one's essential 'humanness', while genuineness is significant in the generation of authenticity: the worker openly providing information requested, and when appropriate initiates information sharing (Kadushin, 1983, p. 65). This involves being honest about the reality of the worker's position: that the worker's powers and limitations are stated clearly when appropriate (Collins and Collins, 1981, p. 34). Authenticity and openness, therefore, involve being authentic as a *professional* and not just a private person. Compton and Galloway (1979, p. 180) incorporate both private and professional persona with genuineness in a form of harmony they call congruence.

> Congruence means that workers bring ... honest openness and realness ... [which] match the underlying value system and essential self as a professional person.

At a personal level it motivates 'a warm and nurturing heart, on objective, open and disciplined mind' (heart and head). It is the *synthesis of personal and professional* which is significant: without this there is 'a loss of spontaneity with the worker appearing as a guarded professional' (Compton and Galloway, 1979, p. 180). For Pippin (1980) this involves an absence of phoniness:

> not taking on the 'air of professionalism' not hiding behind the facade of degrees and credentials (p. 32).

Finally, real genuineness is not possible without a high degree of self under-standing. It is (Perlman, 1979) to be free of pretension ... to have a sense of wholeness ... of knowing who and what one is, what one's guiding values are ... being on fairly good terms with oneself (p. 60)

Nurses' discussion largely mirrors those of social work without, however, discriminating personal and professional genuineness. Barry (1984, p. 141) considers it 'the ability to be human and real in the relationship ... it is ... a sharing of one's self'. Writing influenced by existentialist thought emphasizes nursing as a meeting of persons: they are both subjects with the capabilities for internal relationships and they 'can be open or available and knowable to each other' (Paterson and Zderad, 1976, pp. 26–9). French (1983, p. 175) asserts that the nurse 'cannot be phoney', they must be spontaneous and open, and not hide behind their role as counsellor. They must 'be a human being to the human beings before him'. No mention here of the complexity added by professional responsibility. Tschudin (1987, p. 22) adopts a similar position. There should be a harmony between the inner and outer aspects of the persons, between what we feel and what we say; there should be a large measure of self awareness; but we should not 'take refuge in our perceived role'. Authenticity for Burnard (1985, p. 11) appears similar to Kadushin's perception of genuineness: the authentic person consistently acting in accordance with their own values, wishes and feelings. In truth, authenticity and genuineness may be difficult to distinguish. However, some nurse authors may become confused as are Ward and Bishop (1988, p. 39) between genuineness and acceptance:

Genuineness involves developing respect for that person as an individual ... and unconditionally accepting the person for who he is.

How does the nurse demonstrate genuineness? French (1983, p. 75) suggests the nurse should give time, be sincere and be consistent in the attitudes and behaviour shown during the interview. However sincerity does not involve cushioning the patient inappropriately from reality. Porritt (1984) advocates giving

information which people often shy away from giving to another person who sometimes really wants to know the worst, and other times really wants not to know. (p. 109)

Commitment/Care/Concern for Others

Commitment, care or concern for others is extensively discussed in social work, but less so in nursing literature, although, of course, qualities such as empathy or genuineness presuppose concern. This concern (Perlman, 1979,

p. 59) 'implies ... that one cares about the person's hurt and/or about the hurtful consequences of his behaviour, whether for himself or others'. Perlman here emphasizes that concern is not just for the individual, but more generally for relevant affected others. It involves (Kadushin, 1983, p. 56) 'a sincere interest in the client and his predicament'. Haines (1981, p. 131) believes concern for others to be basic to social work practice: the worker's contribution to the relationship with the client springing from his/her concern for other human beings. Keith-Lucas (1972, pp. 85–7) suggests one aspect is support, which draws attention to another element: the worker will not give up on the client. In particular the client must know they will not be deserted because they in some respect disappoint the worker. Similarly, Compton and Galloway (1979) refer to commitment and obligation: a determination to further clients' interests:

> unqualified by our idiosyncratic personal needs ... a wish to further the purpose of the relationship without the expectation of returns (p. 168).

This can, according to Haines (1981) create an emotional link — bonding — the feeling that someone else, albeit a professional person, has confidence in the client's ability to solve his/her own problems. Care and concern may obviously occur in normal social circumstances, but they may become high level skills (Haines, 1981, pp. 131–2) 'they can be developed and refined to the point where their use becomes a highly skilled operation'. How, though, is concern expressed? It centrally involves the response of the worker to the client — 'by asking ... for his story, his feelings, his reactions, by making replies that indicate how well we have been listening' (Kadushin, 1983, p. 55). Ragg (1977, p. 5) suggests it should be expressed in terms of the client's everday experience rather than technical terms like psychological forces, and presented in everyday language — of experience, bitterness, failure and so on. Pippin (1980) believes caring is largely transmitted non-verbally: the tone of voice, facial expression, gestures used, body posture and so on.

Information/Advice/Social Skills Education

A number of 'expert skills' may be identified. The first, all characterized by the provision of information in one form or another, is a group cluster of information, advice and social skills education. It is important, first, that the worker is *knowledgeable* about the subject matter of the interview. Kadushin (1983, p. 17) argues that knowledge enables the worker to make sense of what he is seeing and hearing, and of relationships between items of information which would escape those ignorant of the subject matter. Information giving is important to social work practice. Anderson (1988, p. 164) thinks it 'is a skill so ubiquitous in social work practice that it is often taken for granted'. Middleman and Goldberg (1974, p. 118), although equally emphatic about its importance, considers it a more discrete activity, appropriate 'if, and only if, the information is relevant to the task in hand and not already available to the other'. Nonetheless, it may occur at any or all points in the social work process, and may cover a wide range of activities: facts, opinions and ideas, increasing knowledge of situations and events. Haines (1981, p. 75) divides information giving into two: factual, to increase knowledge about service availability, and information about how to *set about* achieving an object — e.g. which organization or person is appropriately contacted.

Advice is a closely related activity. Siporin (1975, p. 310) relates advice only to practical issues: the social worker steering or advising the client to apply on his own to another agency. Advice is intended to enable the client rather than the worker to carry out tasks. Haines (1981, p. 76) goes beyond practical concerns, identifying two types: advice on the best way to achieve an object — e.g. contacting a sympathetic rather than unsympathetic councillor; or interpersonal advice about a particular approach to resolve difficulties — e.g. reducing arguments. Kadushin (1983, p. 203) identifies three elements: explicit directions of what the client should or ought to do; suggestions of alternatives for the client's consideration; and questions worded in a manner to point the direction the worker hopes the client will go. Collins and Collins (1981, p. 62) warn it should 'relate to the selection of means rather than goals'. The client here determines the end to be pursued, the worker only the best way to pursue it. Overall, Hollis (1970) calls information *and* advice 'direct influence', which involves a range of techniques aimed at facilitating the client.

Education in social skills — those of everyday life are also considered significant (Haines, 1981, p. 79). They are concerned with learning how to live, to deal effectively with learning how to plan for the future where appropriate to client needs. Germain and Gitterman (1980, p. 53) summarize the role of social skills teacher:

> The social worker carries out the function of teaching adaptive skills
> through clarifying perceptions ... offering advice and suggestions
> ... modelling desired behaviour, and teaching the steps of problem
> solving.

Some nurse authors also identify information and advice. Pepleau (1988) considers nurses have taught much that was necessary for patient and community health and are 'a source of supply on knowledge and technical procedures'. It is important, she thinks, to discriminate between the roles of teacher and counsellor. Nurses must discriminate, she thinks, between questions 'that require direct, straightforward factual answers and ... those that involve feelings and may require application of the principles of counselling'. French (1983, p. 101) also emphasizes information giving, though this very much revolves around the illness. Yet, he suggests, research indicates information giving is one of the most inefficiently used of nursing skills despite being 'frequently best placed as providers of information'. Kagan *et al.* (1986, p. 141) comment that nurses often respond to requests for information with attempts to reassure the patient, which rarely work. They suggest a process, which, however, seems rather laborious. It involves checking the extent of recipients' knowledge, planning, presentation — which should be precise and accurate — and concluding, which may involve summarizing, checking for understanding and so on. One dubious approach promoted in some nursing (though not social work) literature is *persuasion*. Kagan *et al.* (1986) state:

> there are many situations where nurses have to persuade other people about the desirability of doing certain things connected with the illness (p. 181).

and Smith and Bass (1982) advocating the use of persuasion with patients suggest:

> persuasion is a deliberate attempt to change, reinforce or instill beliefs or behaviour by means of one's image or prestige, by reason and by appeals to the emotions. (p. 136)

This sits uneasily with advocacy of counselling. Some methods of influencing are dubious — use of image or prestige, or appeals to the emotions, and such approaches do not facilitate active and willing choice, by which the patient decides, for good or ill, what they want. Rather the attempt is to make them decide what the *nurse* wants. Furthermore, it assumes not only that the nurse knows more or knows best, but that they know better how or what to decide when the evidence is presented.

Expert Skills

Therapeutic Skills

Therapeutic skills are a group designed broadly to develop insight in clients, and to release feelings which enable them to function better. Those identified in social work may be divided into three broad groups. *Clarification* is a process which enables clients to reorder their thinking about themselves and their situation (Haines, 1981). Middleman and Goldberg (1974, p. 122) call this *connecting discrete events*, which are not perceived by clients as connected. It is used when '(1) the worker infers a connection and (2) connecting the events puts a different perspective on the client's plight'. Shulman (1984) identifies two skills contributing to clarification. First, there are *elaborating skills*, when client's presentations are fragmentary, which focus questions to help clients to 'elaborate and clarify specific concerns. Second there is *putting (dimly appreciated) client feelings into words*: 'by articulating this emotion, the worker gives permission to the client to discuss his own feelings about himself'.

A second group of skills are designed to *promote self understanding*, or the discovery of self. Haines (1981, p. 91) calls this insight development which he considers 'an essential element of emotional health'. He considers it a painful and difficult process entailing recognition of aspects of personality often preferable to ignore. Middleman and Goldberg (1974, p. 147) suggest additionally that personal and social taboos exist which protect self from guilt or embarrassment in highly sensitive areas, and these present obstacles to true self understanding and task accomplishment. Hollis (1972) emphasizes this therapy is not simply *internal* but occurs in a *situational context* — it is psychosocial. She identifies three elements: *pattern dynamic reflection* (like exploration of self), reflecting upon internal reasons for behaviour; *person-situation reflection* which involves reflection on the relationship between their internal state and the situational factors confronting them; and *developmental reflection* which concentrates on early life experiences, internalized to become part of his responses to current situations. Siporin (1975, p. 299), like Hollis, sees this as psychosocial. It is not, therefore, just an enhancement of understanding, but it should *help the client change*, thus 'helping him to discover and actualize his creative powers, to realize his capacities and strengths for personal change and growth'.

A third group of skills may broadly be described as *enabling* skills. Enabling skills are those 'carefully guided by the social worker', through which clients become better able to manage their life and problems (Haines, 1981, p. 81). Anderson (1988, p. 64) calls this 'freeing' — assisting, releasing, facilitating and so on — which 'stimulates his or her individual growth process'. This involves, first, *release of feelings*, and clients should understand they can express feelings safely. Hollis (1972) suggests

> the worker encourages the client to ventilate feelings that have been restrained or suppressed . . . feelings of anger or hatred are especially likely to lose some of their intensity. (p. 78)

Sustainment (Hollis, 1972, p. 78) or *encouragement* (Haines, 1981, p. 87) involves building client's strengths, helping people feel better about themselves and provision of reassurance. Another aspect is *confrontation* (Middleman and Goldberg, 1974, p. 148) or *challenge* (Anderson, 1988, p. 119). Where information is skewed or contradictory (in, for example, verbal versus non-verbal information) this can block work on tasks, by preventing discussion of relevant concerns and this may be challenged. Anderson considers this potentially threatening and argues that adequate support is a necessary prerequisite to challenge. The client, furthermore, should only be expected to move step by step rather than a quantum leap in perspective following a challenge.

In the nursing literature, therapeutic skills are discussed mainly in the 'nurse as counsellor' literature. Nurse counselling is defined as 'a therapeutic conversation between two people in an understanding atmosphere' (Burnard, 1985, p. 70) 'a catalyst for self exploration' (Litwack *et al.*, 1980) 'to assist the individual to make his own decisions from among the choices available' (Nurse, 1975, p. 2) 'to give the clear opportunity to explore, discover and clarify ways of living more satisfyingly' (Tschudin, 1987, p. 3). The skills discussed in nursing literature fall primarily into those defined as clarification and, to a lesser degree, enabling. Promotion of self understanding or discovery of self skills are almost entirely absent from the nursing literature, perhaps because of the skills limitations in nurses. These may be the skills of which they are most wary: as Dartington *et al.* (1977) point out, they are not preparing to be counsellors but just to use counselling skills. Indeed Tschudin (1987, p. 3) comments that those who counsel will be 'a nurse with more than the expected skills'.

Clarification skills include *exploration* and analysis through which nurses may 'explore the area surrounding the problem' (Nurse, 1975, p. 59), and which may involve closed or open questions (Marks–Maran, 1988, p. 75). A second involves *reflecting thoughts and feelings* (Kagan *et al.*, 1986). In the process

> the nurse reflects back to the client ... the factual content ... of what he is saying, and ... the feelings as she perceives them. (p. 196)

There are, here, three elements: the factual content, the feelings presented, and the nurses' perceptions which provide a frame for these. Tschudin (1987, p. 86) calls this 'holding up a mirror' to the client (presumably metaphorically). Bridge and Mcleod–Clark (1986, p. 87) suggest repeating the last part of the patients' statement as a question in order to encourage reflection. Paraphrasing is closely associated: Stewart (1983, p. 59) calls this a 'free rendering or an amplification of a statement' aimed at helping those finding difficulty expressing themselves. Nurses may also reflect what is *not* said: 'in reflecting we also respond to the unsaid or unheard, but implied' (Tschudin, 1987, p. 86). A further element is summarizing, through which (Barry, 1984)

> the helper is able to extract the essence of what a patient has intellectually and affectively experienced during their time together. (p. 148)

Tschudin (1987) thinks this can provide direction to scattered thoughts and feelings. A more advanced skill is *interpreting* or *reframing*. This involves giving a client an interpretation of a situation so that he can understand himself better in relation to it (Nurse, 1975; Tschudin, 1987, p. 106). A final element is *focusing* (Barry, 1984, p. 148) 'best used after the client has had a chance to discuss various topics', by which the helper 'zeros' into a specific event of the client's explorations.

Two major *enabling* skills are identified. The first is *catharsis* (or release of feelings) through which the client relieves emotional tension, and which enables the client to gain new insights into his condition, become more spontaneous, and able to take charge of his life (Burnard, 1985, p. 95). *Confronting* is also advocated where appropriate by nurse authors to deal with discrepancies between thought and feeling, what we are and what we think we are (Tschudin, 1987, p. 103) or alternatively where the client is presented with the likely outcome of his behaviour (Stewart, 1983, p. 74). French (1983) likewise advocates appropriate challenging of distortions and discrepancies, but to do so without leaving the client 'feeling trapped'. Barry (1984, p. 109) though adds a cautionary note consistent with earlier statements that 'confronting is a skill that should be used cautiously at this level [i.e. nurse's] of counselling'.

Analytic Processes

Analytic processes is a term to describe the step by step process of rational analysis and intervention evident in both nursing and social work literature. In social work, these are broadly divided into Assessment; Planning and Goal Setting; Intervention Tasks; and Ending and Evaluation. A key element is *client participation*, and this is particularly evident with contracting. Hence, Collins and Collins (1981, p. 1) consider success 'demands the maximum degree of collaboration and mutual understanding between client and worker'. Contracts are often considered the way to achieve this, involving 'a shared definition of the problem and an explicit mutual agreement about their goals, tasks, respective roles and terms of work' (Germain and Gitterman, 1980, p. 53). Haines (1981, p. 209) likewise writes of 'explicit consensual agreements'. Corden and Preston-Shoot (1987, p. x) agree and suggest that 'social workers do not necessarily know best', while Hollis (1970, p. 57) pragmatically considers it 'irresponsible' not to enlist the client's involvement.

Assessment aims (Collins and Collins, 1981, p. 18) 'to arrive ... at the best possible understanding of his situation ... [as] a basis for helping him resolve his problems.' It has been divided (though not always) into social study — the identification of the psychosocial and environmental elements of the client's situation (Siporin, 1975, p. 220) and diagnosis, the 'process of discovering patterns of significance' (Sainsbury, 1970, p. 17) or 'the effort to deduce from the material available ... what the client's trouble is' (Hollis, 1970, p. 49). More recently authors have been unhappy with the use of a term derived from medicine, instead preferring the general term assessment, or, as with Ragg (1977, p. 78), description. Although important at the outset, Shulman (1984, p. 209) emphasizes assessment should be a continuous process throughout intervention. *Planning* has been defined as a 'deliberate rational process that involves the choice of actions that are calculated to achieve specific objectives' (Gurin, 1972, p. 49). Goals 'make explicit what the practitioner and client expect to accomplish ... the desired state ... to work toward' (Reid, 1978, p. 34), although Epstein (1985, p. 68) distinguishes agency, professional, personal practitioner and client goals, which *may* differ. Hollis (1970, p. 57) also distinguishes between ultimate goals, which may be quite general at the outset, and proximate goals, for the immediate future, which should be clear and specific. Reid (1978, p. 92) suggests the central question for the plan is 'what can be done to alleviate the client's difficulties?' and suggests three significant factors: action requirements, obstacles (barriers susceptible to alteration) and constraints (limits to action alternatives). Epstein (1985, p. 272) identifies a number of elements to the plan: defining the change target, identifying goals, choosing intervention activities, and formulating a sequence. *Intervention* tasks are discussed in detail by Reid (1978, p. 139): they are 'the central problem solving actions the client or practitioner agree to undertake'. These are the outcome of the planning process, and it is important to recognize that tasks should be precise and undertaken in the appropriate sequence. In addition to client tasks there are practitioner's tasks which may be facilitative — to help the client carry out their tasks — or independent tasks, which are entirely separate. Finally, Reid (1978) refers to *endings*, which involve *evaluation*. This has two elements: first the assessment of what has been achieved in relation to target problems, particularly compared with the situation at the outset, and second it involves the client's own conception of change, including change in other areas of the client's life.

There is some ambivalence in the nursing literature about *patient involvement*, which may reflect the interpersonal versus patient centred orientations. McFarlane and Castledene (1982) hardly consider patient participation in their analysis of the nurse process. The most the nurse offers is information (rather than participation) because

> he has a right to know what is *going to happen to himself* [my italics] as
> a result he is more likely to co-operate. (p. 58)

Likewise, Marks–Maran (1988, p. 82) states 'day to day care planning requires *nurses* [my italics] to select what is right or wrong in nursing care'. Others, however, emphasize patient involvement. Pepleau (1988, p. 23) suggests engaging 'him as an active partner'. Others agree (French, 1983, p. 16; Smith and Bass, 1982, p. 209; Bottorff and D'Cruz, 1984) and Yuen (1984, p. 532) emphasizes 'the client should not be provided with ready made decisions, but encouraged to find a solution to his own problems.'

The phases of the nursing process resemble the social work literature analyzed. *Assessment* for D'arcy (1984, p. 72) is 'obtaining information and conducting a critical assessment to identify problems which may be resolved in nursing care'. This involves a review of information and a comparison, in terms of daily living activities, of patient functioning with normal physiological, psychological and social functioning (McFarlane and Castledene,

1982, p. 17) and involves both the patient and their situation. French (1983, p. 18), Smith and Bass (1982, p. 199) call this the 'analysis stage': it involves identifying the problem and analyzing it to understand its nature, scope and sub-problem. Diagnosis (Marks–Maran, 1988, p. 54) 'identifies the problems or unmet needs which a patient has'. *Planning*, according to Ritter (1989, p. 13) has two components: formulating specific problems out of situations and the statement of objectives designed to improve or resolve two elements to objectives: a definition of situation and goals and consideration of various strategies available to achieve the goals. Smith and Bass (1982, p. 197) suggest three elements to strategies: determining alternative solutions, determining the criteria by which solutions may be evaluated, and evaluating the alternatives in terms of these criteria, through which the best strategy is chosen.

Implementation is the next stage in the process.

> To implement is to carry out the interventions required to achieve the objectives stated in nursing care plans. (Ritter, 1989, p. 13)

It involves a number of considerations: the ability of the patient to care for themselves; various categories of action (manual, counselling, information, communication and teaching skills); providing a physical and psychological environment for care (McFarlane and Castledene, 1982, p. 89). The 'expected outcome' are objectives or goals 'comprising outcomes defined in the planning stage' (Ritter, 1989, p. 28) or 'whether they are meeting stated goals' (D'arcy, 1984, p. 79). Kagan *et al.* (1986, p. 170) emphasize (like Reid, 1978) that *evaluation* is not simply the last stage of the intervention process; it should occur at various points during this process.

Comments

A number of conclusions derive from this analysis. First, where interpersonal or relationship elements of practice are discussed in social work and nursing they possess, if not a common language in detail, common areas of interest. However, while in social work relationship skills are considered fundamental and provide a 'glue' which binds together disparate areas of practice, there is an ambivalence in nursing between the interpersonal and more patient (i.e. medical) orientations of practice. As these are not complementary, there is some feeling that the latter may actually impede the former. There is, furthermore, no reason to consider, despite its area of interest, that psychiatric nursing is any more advanced in this respect than other areas of nursing. The psychiatric nursing literature does not display a more sophisticated understanding of interpersonal processes or skills. Indeed many of the basic texts show a complete absence of awareness of, or merely a passing reference to, the importance of these skills. Even where these skills are examined in nursing literature, their approach is rather fragmentary. The reader is confronted with different areas: communication skills for nursing, nursing as an interpersonal process, or counselling skills for nurses. These contrast with social work, where the equivalent of all these for social work are examined in text with titles which revealingly imply coherence and unity (e.g. *Skills and Method in Social Work*, (Haines); *Foundations of Social Work Practice*, (Anderson).

Furthermore, even where these skills are examined in nursing it is at times undertaken in a half hearted manner. A number of nurse authors warn nurses about handling counselling skills with care — nurses can be expected only to have limited skills of this sort. There is a noticeable absence, compared with social work literature of skills related to the promotion of self understanding, which may be considered particularly difficult (and dangerous) to handle. Even some nursing literature actually examining interpersonal and nursing processes present analysis which is superficial in the extreme. Thus Burnard (1985) for example, suggests that

> warmth, transparency (or openness) and genuineness are self explanatory ... unconditional positive regard is the quality of totally respecting the work of the person. (p. 70)

Here we have a number of concepts raised, defined (in one case) and dismissed. However, some discussions may even be dangerous. Empathy, for McFarlane and Castledene (1982) involves responding in a way

> that conveys sympathy [???] and understanding so that the patient feels secure and encouraged.... Examples of empathic responses are 'that must have upset you' or 'how difficult it must have been for you'.

This can be dangerously simplistic or patronizing. One can only imagine the response of a woman whose infant has been a cot death to 'that must have upset you' or 'how difficult it must have been for you'. If she had the strength she might be inclined to punch the nurse in the face!

Although, finally, both social work and nursing literature examine common areas — genuineness, empathy, communication, etc. the skills in these are operationalized rather better in social work. Hence Middleman and Goldberg (1974, p. 85) in the area of 'engaging feelings' describe various processes: reaching for feelings, waiting out feelings, getting with feelings, reporting own feelings and reaching for a feeling link. Likewise, Shulman (1984, p. 77ff.) in the area of 'demand for work skills' identifies partializing client concerns, holding to focus, checking for underlying ambivalence and challenging the illusion of work. If nurses are to access anything approaching this, it would require using counselling rather than nursing literature.

Chapter 7

Clients' and Workers' Views of Intervention

Client studies have not played a major part in British mental health research. Brandon (1981) has pointed to the active resistance by some to accepting the views of people labelled mad or disturbed apart from confirming diagnosis. Clients are expected to play a passively responsive role as they experience the skilled help of mental health professionals. What might be termed the arrogance of psychiatry has not been duplicated in social work, where there have been many consumer studies (Fisher, 1983; Rees and Wallace, 1982).

Analysis of client views was undertaken in a series of interviews and in two parts: the first qualitative and the second quantitative. The quantitative part was undertaken on a form designed to reflect, in many areas, precisely the categories available in relation to the workers. Hence these were identical in relation to social and physical ill health problems and activities undertaken. Additional information, also identical to the workers' questionnaire included problems tackled, intervention effect and most effective activity. Further information was elicited in relation to the focus for intervention and client participation in identifying and resolving problems. Altogether seventy-seven clients were interviewed: thirty-eight, evenly divided between CPNs and social workers, who received extended intervention, and thirty-nine, evenly distributed between CPN, social work and joint clients who received extended intervention (see Appendix 1).

This chapter, then, attempts to examine a number of issues generated by the discussion on worker client relationships. First worker client communication is examined through the likely effect of good communication — client awareness of worker definitions of problems and intervention. It is assumed that where communication is good clients will be more accurately aware of workers' definitions. Second, the extent mutual agreement (between client and worker) in problem definition, is analyzed through concordance and discordance between client and worker. Third, the extent to which clients would have preferred alternative or additional work to be undertaken (and hence by implication deficiencies in intervention) is examined. Fourth, the extent to which clients agreed with workers' assessment of change is analyzed. Finally, the degree to which the client felt responsible for the problems themselves, and also the part they played in the process of tackling them, is examined.

Satisfaction

One generally used measure in relation to clients is that of satisfaction. On its own this tells us only a small amount about the client's experience. Fisher (1983, p. 40) identifies a number of problems with this concept. First, he suggests that merely asking people to rate something usually produces favourable evaluations. Second clients may pronounce themselves satisfied knowing little about the alternative services available to them. Third, satisfaction may relate to the *way* a service is given rather than the adequacy of the service itself. This can mean that ratings of satisfaction are not necessarily related to outcome: clients may pronounce themselves satisfied without improvements occuring. Fisher (1983, p. 41) comments:

> ultimately, then, the emphasis on the concept of satisfaction gives us only a very crude understanding of the reaction of clients ... client satisfaction is just one item of information among many which are taken into account when reviewing ... services.

Analysis of satisfaction, therefore, has limitations. It is a very general concept which gives us little detail about the nuances of intervention. However, it provides a useful starting point if used simply to identify — as it was in this case — a general sense of whether the client on the whole felt positively or negatively about intervention. It is supplemented by a detailed analysis of a whole series of factors which examine the clients' experience of intervention and their evaluation of outcome.

The clients were asked to indicate their level of satisfaction on a five point scale from very satisfied to very dissatisfied (table 7.1). There was a noticeable tendency for clients receiving extended intervention to be more positive than those receiving brief intervention, both overall and comparing the individual (CPN and social work) client groups. This may well reflect the outcome of intervention: the greater length of involvement helping create greater positive change. Additionally, however, longer involvement may encourage a relationship through which the client feels more reluctant to criticize the worker. The mere fact that the client gets to know the worker and identifies positive personal qualities may make criticism more difficult to present. Although differences do not reach significance, a comparison of occupation groups shows CPN clients consistently to be less satisfied and more dissatisfied than either social work or joint clients. The data for extended social work intervention are particularly interesting: 85 per cent were satisfied and over half were very satisfied with the help they received. While

Table 7.1   Client Satisfaction

| | BRIEF | | | | | | | | EXTENDED | | | |
| | Social Work | | CPN | | Joint | | Total | | Social | | CPN | |
	No.	%	No.	%	No.	%	No.	%	No.	%	No.	%
Very satisfied	5	39	1	8	4	31	10	26	10	53	7	37
Quite satisfied	3	23	4	31	4	31	11	28	6	32	8	42
Neither satisfied nor dissatisfied	3	23	4	31	3	22	10	26	2	11	1	5
Quite dissatisfied	2	15	1	8	1	8	4	10	—	—	1	5
Very dissatisfied	—	—	3	23	1	8	4	10	1	5	2	11
			P = 0.5326						P = 0.2649			

Table 7.2   Client Agreement with Workers' Definitions of Primary Problem

| | BRIEF | | | | | | | | EXTENDED | | | | | |
| | Social Work | | CPN | | Joint | | Total | | Social Work | | CPN | | Total | |
	No.	%	No.	%	No.	%	No.	%	No.	%	No.	%	No.	%
Mental Health														
Agreed	5	100	4	57	4	80	13	76	2	40	6	50	8	47
Disagreed	0	—	3	43	1	20	4	24	3	60	6	50	9	53
Social														
Agreed	7	88	5	83	4	50	16	73	6	43	4	57	10	48
Disagreed	1	12	1	17	4	50	6	27	8	57	3	43	11	52
TOTAL AGREED	12	92	9	69	8	62	29	74	8	42	10	53	18	47
			P = 0.1741						P = 0.6248					

the overall low levels of dissatisfaction by client groups for both brief and extended intervention are interesting, it is worth noting that the clients interviewed were voluntary clients (as opposed to clients who are required to receive intervention, as with some child care), and might be expected to be more positive than clients who are non-voluntary.

Problems

Clients' perceptions of primary problems were compared with those of the worker in order to identify the number of occasions they agreed with the worker and when they disagreed. The results show a number of interesting trends, although differences are not statistically significant. First, there is a markedly higher agreement between worker and clients receiving brief intervention than those receiving extended intervention. This is perhaps surprising: extended intervention provides the opportunity for lengthier communication with the client and worker clarifying and agreeing about the main problem. Indeed extended intervention was characterized slightly more by disagreement than agreement. Certainly it is interesting that intervention can occur over an extended period of time with predominantly satisfied clients without, in a majority of cases, agreement occurring between client and worker on the primary problems. Brief intervention, on the other hand, was characterized by a relatively high overall agreement between worker and client both in relation to mental health and social primary problems. It may be that, with brief intervention, the workers had less opporunity for detailed assessment. As a result, in some cases the workers may have had to rely to a greater degree on the client's own definition of their primary problem. Comparison of occupations also show distinct trends, varying between brief and extended intervention. With brief intervention social workers and their clients were far more likely to agree about the primary problem than either CPN or joint workers. However, with extended intervention CPNs were more likely to agree with their clients than social workers. It appears from this that CPNs may have been slightly better than social workers at making use of the opportunity for joint problem agreement with clients provided by extended intervention.

These data, although divided up into mental health and social problem areas represent correlations of individual categories within these areas. Thus, for example, depression was correlated with depression, marital problems with marital problems and so on. An alternative way of correlating would be to do so in terms of broad problem areas: neurotic, psychiatric and alcohol or drug abuse within mental health, and practical, emotional and relationship and physical ill health within the social/health problem area. If this is undertaken, the situation changes markedly with extended intervention: both CPNs and social work clients agreed on eleven and disagreed on eight occasions with their worker. Hence workers and clients were operating at times with definitions in the same broad problem areas even when they disagreed on the precise nature of the problem. It is worth noting that clients appeared less comfortable when discussing mental health problems, and this is likely to have had some impact on the results (discussed below and in the Appendix 1). With extended intervention social work clients identified depression as the primary problem on five occasions. On four of these occasions social workers identified emotional problems as primary. These may reflect different ways of defining the same thing. A client may consider themselves depressed, but the worker, while recognizing the client's depressed feelings may consider it sub-clinical and hence define it as an emotional problem. Interestingly, however, this did not occur with brief intervention, although the level of agreement in general was rather higher.

Table 7.3 shows the concordance and discordance between workers and clients in the identification of mental health problems. This is slightly different from the previous table. Table 7.2 identified the frequency with which clients agreed with the workers' definition of primary problem. Here,

Table 7.3   Mental Health Problems: Concordance and Discordance between Client and Worker

| | BRIEF | | | | | | EXTENDED | | | |
| | Social Worker | | CPN | | Joint | | Social Worker | | CPN | |
	T	%	T	%	T	%	T	%	T	%
Depression	4	25	4	25	5	40	14	29	10	30
Anxiety	5	60	2	50	3	67	2	0	12	42
Phobic	—	—	—	—	—	—	—	—	1	0
Schizophrenia	—	—	—	—	—	—	1	0	—	—
Alcohol abuse	2	100	3	100	2	100	1	0	1	100
Drug abuse	—	—	1	100	—	—	—	—	—	—
Total	11	55	10	60	10	60	18	22	24	38

(T = total number of instances of concordance and discordance
(% = proportion of total instances of concordance and discordance which were concordant)

however, concordance occurred where worker and client identified the same mental health problem, but disconcordance occurred either where the worker identified a mental health problem which the client did not *or* vice versa. This then allows us to compare on equal terms competing definitions (by worker and client) rather than measuring agreement against one group's (the workers') definition. Although both worker and client could only identify one mental health problem, five permutations were possible:

1   Neither worker nor client identified a mental health problem.
2   Both worker and client identified the same mental health problem.
3   The worker identified a mental health problem and the client did not.
4   The client identified a mental health problem and the worker did not.
5   Worker and client identified different mental health problems.

Table 7.3 includes only cases where either worker or client identified a mental health problem (i.e. excluding (1) above).

These data reveal again the perhaps surprising trend that concordance was greater with brief than extended work — indeed quite markedly so. Furthermore, while data for occupations providing brief intervention are practically identical, concordance was noticeably higher between CPNs and their clients than social workers and their clients with extended work. Some care, however, should be taken when interpreting these results. Clients were less comfortable defining mental health problems — some of the terminology such as schizophrenia appearing rather too technical for them — than social problems. This issue is discussed elsewhere (in Appendix 1) but it is likely that some of the discordance arose because of client lack of familiarity with psychiatric terminology. If, as with the primary problem, we correlate additionally workers' identification of emotional problems with client definition

Table 7.4 *Social Problem — proportion of all instances of concordance and discordance in which concordance occurred between client and worker*

| | BRIEF | | | | | | | | EXTENDED | | | | | |
| | Social Work | | CPN | | Joint | | Total | | Social Work | | CPN | | Total | |
	T	%	T	%	T	%	T	%	T	%	T	%	T	%
Practical	11	27	21	23	13	46	45	31	31	52	30	40	61	46
Emotional and relationship	35	66	38	37	35	54	108	52	70	73	57	46	127	61
Ill health	5	60	6	0	7	29	18	28	19	5	25	4	44	2
TOTAL	51	57	65	29	55	49	171	44	120	57	112	35	232	46

(T = total number of instances of concordance and discordance)
(% = Proportion of total instances of concordance and discordance were concordant).

of depression and anxiety, the picture changes dramatically. Concordance between social workers and clients receiving brief intervention occurred in three out of four instances of depression, and four out of five instances of anxiety. CPNs and their clients were concordant in two out of four instances of depression while anxiety showed no change. Joint workers were concordant with their clients in four out of five instances of depression and all three instances of anxiety. Extended intervention reveals still more marked changes. Social workers and clients were concordant with their clients in eight out of ten instances of depression and nine out of twelve instances of anxiety. The effect on overall data is marked (figures presented as per cent of total).

| | *Brief* | | | *Extended* | |
Social Work	*CPN*	*Joint*		*Social Worker*	*CPN*
83	70	90		89	75

The inclusion of workers' data on emotional problems, therefore, indicates high overall levels of concordance. It also indicates clients' concordance with social workers to be higher than that with CPNs.

Concordance and discordance was also examined in relation to social and health problems (table 7.4). As with the workers' questionnaire it was possible for the clients to identify more than one social problem. Each of these broad problem areas represent an aggregation of all instances of concordance and discordance in relation to specific problem categories within each broad area. Hence practical includes financial, housing, home management, etc. Overall, there were small differences between brief and extended intervention in the degree of concordance although extended intervention involved more problems and less concordance with ill health. Social workers, furthermore, showed greater concordance with their clients' views, with both

Table 7.5   Proportion of occasions workers identified mental health problems was accurately identified by clients

	BRIEF								EXTENDED					
	Social Work		CPN		Joint		Total		Social Work		CPN		Total	
	T	%	T	%	T	%	T	%	T	%	T	%	T	%
Depression	2	50	2	0	3	33	7	29	4	100	5	60	9	78
Anxiety	5	0	2	0	2	0	9	0	1	0	11	45	12	42
Alcohol abuse	3	67	3	100	2	100	8	88	1	100	1	100	2	100
Drug abuse	—	—	1	100	—	—	1	100	—	—	—	—	—	—
Schizophrenia	—	—	—	—	—	—	—	—	1	0	—	—	1	0
TOTAL	10	30	8	50	7	43	25	40	7	71	17	53	24	58
			p = 0.6792								p = 0.7043			

(T = total number of cases where workers identified a mental health problem)
(% = proportion of total identified accurately by the client)

brief and extended intervention, than CPN or joint workers. With the exception of ill health both CPNs and social workers showed greater concordance with their clients with extended work, particularly high with social work identification of emotional and relationship problems. This suggests, unlike the levels of agreement on primary problems, that extended work did offer the opportunity for greater mutual agreement over problem definition. This is reflected in detailed analysis. Concordance occurred between social worker and client with extended intervention in all nineteen instances of emotional problems, in ten out of fifteen loss or separation problems, and six out of seven child care problems. Concordance was highest for CPNs with emotional problems (twelve out of eighteen) instances, housing (three out of four) and loss (four out of seven). With brief intervention concordance was highest between social workers and clients with marital problems (all six instances), social relations (seven out of ten instances) and emotional problems (six out of nine instances). Concordance was highest for joint workers with emotional problems (six out of twelve instances), loss/separation (four out of six) and marital problems (three out of five).

A further indication of the quality of communication between worker and client was the extent to which the clients were aware of the workers' perception of their problems. If they were communicating well the worker would be expected to indicate to the client how they defined their problems — indeed they might reach a mutual definition of their problems. This is an approach advocated in much of the social work literature: client involvement in deciding the goals of work, what *they* wish to achieve, and what processes are required to achieve their goals. It is in particular characteristic of approaches involving contracts (Reid, 1978; Corden and Preston-Shoot, 1987). To what extent, then, were clients able accurately to identify workers' perceptions of their mental health problems? Table 7.5 shows the proportion

Table 7.6   Clients' awareness of workers' views of their social problems

| | BRIEF | | | | | | | | EXTENDED | | | | | |
| | Social Work | | CPN | | Joint | | Total | | Social Work | | CPN | | Total | |
	T	%	T	%	T	%	T	%	T	%	T	%	T	%
Practical	5	40	9	44	6	83	20	55	25	52	22	23	47	38
Emotional and relationship	24	88	20	45	28	39	72	57	60	83	34	73	94	78
Ill health	5	60	4	50	1	0	10	50	5	40	2	0	7	29
TOTAL	34	76	33	33	35	35	102	56	90	72	58	52	148	64

(T = total number of cases in which social problems were identified)
(% = Proportion of these identified accurately by the client)

of cases in which clients accurately indicated the workers' view. Again although not statistically significant these data show the greater accuracy of extended clients' perceptions. Indeed under half of the brief clients were accurately aware of workers' definitions. Analysis of client groups also display differences between brief and extended intervention. Social work clients were the least accurate of the three brief client groups, yet they were noticeably more successful than CPNs with extended intervention. Clients receiving brief intervention from all occupation groups were, interestingly, rarely able accurately to identify neurotic problems (depression and anxiety), although there was far greater accuracy with drug and alcohol abuse. Rather greater success in relation to neurotic problems was identified by clients receiving extended intervention, particularly those of social workers.

Table 7.6 shows the client's awareness of workers' views of their problems. These are presented in terms of the number of individual social problems identified within each of the three broad areas. As with mental health problems clients were more accurately aware of worker defined social problems with extended than brief intervention. This is consistent with other data, except for primary problems. It may be that where more complex multi-problems were concerned, the number of problems may have served to obscure clients' awareness of workers' definition of primary problems. With both brief and extended intervention clients were more aware of workers' definition of emotional and relationship problems: indeed the accuracy was particularly high with extended intervention. Social work clients were markedly more able to identify accurately the workers' views of their problems. Detailed analysis of brief intervention shows social work clients to have most accurately identified marital problems (on all six occasions), loss or separation (on all three occasions), social relations and or isolation (six out of seven) and emotional problems (five out of six). CPN clients were most accurate with housing, financial, loss or separation and major illness problems (two out of three occasions for each of these). Joint clients were most accurate with housing and financial problems (two out of two occasions for

Table 7.7   Clients' awareness of problems tacked by workers

| | BRIEF | | | | | | | | EXTENDED | | | | | |
| | Social Work | | CPN | | Joint | | Total | | Social Work | | CPN | | Total | |
	T	%	T	%	T	%	T	%	T	%	T	%	T	%
Practical	1	0	5	20	2	50	8	38	18	39	18	28	36	33
Emotional and relationship	20	65	15	20	16	44	51	45	46	63	29	59	75	61
Ill health	2	0	—	—	2	50	4	25	—	—	1	0	1	0
TOTAL	23	57	20	20	20	45	63	40	64	57	48	46	112	48

(T = total problems tackled; % = proportion accurately identified by client)

each) and loss or separation (three out of five occasions). Social work clients were significantly more able to identify marital (p = 0.05) and social relation or isolation problems (p = 0.0346).[1] Detailed examination of extended work shows social work clients to be most accurate about emotional problems (all nineteen occasions), child care (all six occasions), marital (seven out of eight) and loss or separation problems (nine out of eleven). CPN clients were most accurate about loss or separation (four out of four), emotional (eleven out of twelve) and marital problems (six out of nine).

Perception of Problems Tackled

Intervention

Table 7.7 shows clients' awareness of the problems workers considered themselves to have tackled. Clients were slightly less aware of problems tackled with brief than extended intervention. They were also rather less aware of practical problems tackled than emotional and relationship problems. Clients were generally able to identify less than half the occasions when problems were tackled by workers. The exception to this is social work clients of whom nearly three fifths of problems tackled were accurately identified with both brief and extended intervention. Indeed, social work clients were again more successful than other clients, both with brief and extended work, in identifying problems tackled. More detailed analysis of problem categories shows brief social work clients to be more accurate in identifying marital problems (five out of six occasions), social relations and isolation (four out of seven) and emotional problems tackled (three out of five). CPN clients were most accurate with social relations and isolation (two out of seven) and accurately identified the one housing problem tackled. Joint clients likewise identified the one housing problem tackled, and marital, loss or separation and major illness problems were each identified on one of two occasions tackled. Extended social work clients were most accurate with

Table 7.8   Extent to which client identified activities undertaken by workers

| | BRIEF | | | | | | | | EXTENDED | | | | | |
| | Social Work | | CPN | | Joint | | Total | | Social Work | | CPN | | Total | |
	T	%	T	%	T	%	T	%	T	%	T	%	T	%
Assessor	10	90	8	63	9	78	27	78	19	100	13	92	32	97
Psychosocial treatment and support agent	8	88	7	100	6	83	21	90	44	59	22	68	66	62
Teacher/counsellor	16	56	19	37	17	53	52	48	36	67	32	47	68	57
Broker/advocate	2	50	2	50	1	0	5	40	11	45	1	100	12	42
TOTAL	36	72	36	55	33	67	105	65	110	67	68	62	178	65

(T = total number of activities, as derfined by workers, undertaken within each role area)
(% = the proportion of these activities accurately identified by clients)

emotional problems (fifteen out of nineteen), child care (three out of four) and marital problems (five out of eight). CPN clients were most accurate with emotional problems (nine out of ten) and loss or separation (three out of four).

The clients were, with one exception (brief CPN intervention) able overall to identify above 60 per cent of workers' activities (table 7.8). Interestingly, they were as successful with brief intervention as extended intervention. In other respects the pattern is again similar to other data: social work — and joint — clients were generally able to identify the activities undertaken by their workers more successfully than CPN clients. This was a consistent pattern in activities across all role areas, with the exception of psychosocial treatment and support agent, where CPN clients were more accurate in relation to both brief and extended work. Clients were on the whole, however, most successful overall in identifying the assessment and psychosocial treatment and support agent roles and least accurate with the broker-advocate role. The latter is perhaps not surprising — this role involves advocacy and resource mobilizing, and much of the work will have taken place with agencies and professionals outside face-to-face contact with the client. Detailed analysis of brief intervention shows social work clients to be most accurate in identifying assessment (nine out of ten occasions), ventilation-emotional support (seven out of eight) and discussing future options (seven out of eleven). CPN clients were most accurate with ventilation-emotional support (seven out of seven occasions) and assessment (five out of eight), while joint clients were most accurate with assessment (seven out of nine), ventilation-emotional support (five out of six) and information and advice (four out of seven). Analysis of extended intervention shows social work clients to be most accurate with assessment (all nineteen occasions), ventilation-emotional support (seventeen out of eighteen), and discussing future options (sixteen out of eighteen). CPN clients were most accurate with assessment and ventilation-emotional support (both twelve out of thirteen). There was less agreement over which was the most *effective* activity undertaken. Clients receiving brief intervention agreed with the worker on only three out of thirteen cases for each occupation group. Both CPN and joint clients agreed with the worker only in relation to ventilation-emotional support (three occasions each) while social work clients agreed on one case each of information and advice, advocacy and ventilation-emotional support. With extended intervention clients agreed with the worker more frequently, although even this was more frequent amongst social work clients (nine or 47 per cent of cases) then CPN clients (six or 32 per cent of cases). Agreement between social worker and client occurred four out of five times with psychosocial work, four out of seven times with ventilation-emotional support and once out of five instances of psychosocial work, and the one instance of social skills education.

Clients were also asked whether there were some activities they would like to have had undertaken by the worker, but which did not in fact take place: that is, were they satisfied that the work undertaken was all that it could have been to help them? Although this does not mean that activities actually undertaken were not appreciated, it provides some indication of the perceived adequacy of intervention. Again the CPNs fared poorest in this respect. With brief intervention only three (23 per cent) social work and four (31 per cent) joint clients compared with nine (69 per cent) CPN clients wished for some alternative activities (p = 0.0374). Only three (16 per cent) social work clients compared with ten (53 per cent) CPN clients receiving extended intervention wanted some alternative activity (p = 0.0402). Over half of all CPN clients, therefore, considered the work undertaken to be deficient in some respect. The deficiencies identified most frequently by brief CPN clients were discussing future options and social skills education (three occasions each) information and advice, psychodynamic work, and advocacy (two cases of each). Some of these, such as psychodynamic work and social skills education imply the need for more extended intervention. Clients of joint workers identified psychodynamic work on three occasions with similar implications. With extended work, CPN clients most frequently identified psychodynamic work (five cases) and discussing future options (three cases); on two occasions social work clients also identified psycho-dynamic work. This emphasis on the deficiency in psychodynamic work by CPNs reflects its (relatively) low frequency in the analysis of extended intervention (Chapter 5).

Clients were also asked what they felt was the main focus for intervention. This choices were the client alone, client and spouse or family, client plus acquaintances or friends, spouse or family, acquaintances or friends, group or outside agencies. They generally identified the client alone as the main focus. This was the case for eleven social work and ten CPN and joint clients (respectively) receiving brief intervention. The rest identified the client plus spouse or family to be the main focus. With extended intervention sixteen (out of nineteen) of both CPN and social work clients considered the client to be the main focus. Three social work clients identified groupwork and the three CPNs clients identified the client plus spouse or family. The clients were also asked if they would have preferred an alternative focus: all three social work clients receiving groupwork would have preferred the primary focus to be on them alone, while two CPN clients preferred a focus to be on the spouse, family, friends or acquaintances (the other wanted the focus on him/herself). Client perception of the appropriate focus was predominantly therefore on themselves. This would, of course, largely reflect their experience of intervention. Furthermore, focusing on them may for many clients mean making their interests of central importance. This would not necessarily preclude work with outside groups or agencies.

Clients were asked whether or not the development of their problems were largely out of their control, and to what extent they were involved in the management of their problems. Of clients receiving brief work, four social work (31 per cent), three CPN (23 per cent) and five joint clients felt they bore some responsibility for their problems. Five CPN and social work clients respectively (26 per cent) receiving extended intervention also felt some responsibility. Client involvement in the management of their problems was analyzed in terms of work mainly undertaken by the client, mainly undertaken by the worker or equal responsibility. The tasks were divided up into defining the problem(s), planning intervention, and tasks aimed at resolution or amelioration of problems. The problems themselves were divided up into practical/financial, child care/familial, other social network relations, personal functioning and physical ill health. Work undertaken mainly by the worker was rare with brief intervention. Social work clients felt problems were defined in this way only twice, while planning and task performance were carried out mainly by the worker on seven and one occasions respectively. CPN and joint clients both identified only four problem areas where planning was undertaken mainly by the worker. In the majority of instances the client felt it was mainly they who defined problems, planned and carried out tasks to manage the problems. Social work clients identified ninety-four instances of defining, planning and carrying out tasks of which eighty-one were undertaken mainly by the client. This was the case with CPN clients in ninety out of ninety-four instances and for joint workers in sixty-two out of sixty-nine instances across all problem areas. Overwhelmingly, therefore, the clients saw themselves as most significant in defining, planning and task performance. Extended work showed a different pattern. Social work clients considered 19 per cent of instances of defining planning and task performing was mainly undertaken by the worker; in 27 per cent they considered this to be equal and in 54 per cent of instances mainly the client (total 156 instances). Of 147 instances cited by CPN clients, 11 per cent were mainly undertaken by the worker, 22 per cent were equal and 67 per cent were mainly undertaken by the client. Clearly clients overall saw themselves taking the bulk of responsibility in dealing with their problems. However extended intervention involved greater emphasis on the worker's contribution, not surprising perhaps given the greater opportunity for workers to influence the intervention process. Finally, with extended intervention, social workers on balance exerted more influence on matters. This is interesting, for on one hand this might be intrepreted as CPNs being less directive and allowing clients room to make their own decisions, while on the other hand social workers might be seen to be providing more positive input to help clients. The details of clients' views of this will be examined in later chapters.

Clients were also asked how open they felt workers were in saying what they were thinking and doing in relation to various problems. CPNs were considered not open more frequently than social workers, although the differences were marginal; with brief intervention one social work (8 per cent) and two CPN, but no joint, clients considered their worker not to be open in one of the problem areas with extended intervention; one social work (5 per cent) and three CPN (16 per cent) clients considered them not to be open with extended work. With brief intervention CPNs were considered not open in two instances of practical functioning problems; social workers were also considered not open in one personal functioning and one social network problem. With extended work CPNs were considered not open in two instances of child care and family problems and one personal functioning. Social workers were considered not to be open with one practical problem. Overwhelmingly, therefore, clients considered their workers to be open in their dealings.

Index of Change

Interviews with clients offered the opportunity to compare the workers' view of change with that of the clients. Clients' perceptions of change were calculated in exactly the same way as that shown in Chapters 4 and 5. Table 7.9 shows the *difference*, positive or negative, between clients' and workers' perceptions of change. It should be noted here that, as workers and clients often define different problems, they will, at times be indicating change in relation to different problems. However, the overall index of change nonetheless allows comparison of the degree of change defined by the client, in problems defined by the client, with that defined by the worker. The data presented relate, of course, only to those cases where clients were interviewed.

These data are striking. In relation to mental health problems, social work and joint clients were more positive about change through brief intervention than the workers themselves. Indeed this relates also to extended social work intervention. This process is most marked with brief social work, in particular with neurotic problems. The reverse was the case with CPNs, whose clients were noticeably less positive about intervention than

Table 7.9   Index of Change — differences between client and work perceptions

| | **BRIEF** | | | **EXTENDED** | |
	Social Work	CPN	Joint	Social Work	CPN
Neurotic	+0.4250	−0.333	+0.244	+0.267	−0.592
Psychotic	—	—	—	—	—
Alcohol and drug abuse	0.0000	−0.250	+1.000	−0.000	−1.000
Overall mental health	+0.330	−0.286	+0.257	+0.241	−0.618
Practical	+0.150	−0.317	+0.014	0.000	−0.389
Emotional/relationship	−0.123	−0.514	+0.147	−0.308	−0.356
Ill health	0.000	0.000	+0.500	−0.333	−0.952
Overall social	−0.013	−0.475	+0.024	−0.300	−0.532

the CPNs themselves. This was most markedly the case with brief intervention with neurotic problems. The situation is rather different with social problem change. Only clients of joint workers receiving brief intervention were consistently more positive about change than workers. In no area were brief CPN clients more positive than their worker, and social work clients were consistently (except social work with practical problems) less positive than their workers. However, CPN clients consistently, with both brief and extended intervention, displayed a wider 'negative gap' between themselves and their workers than social work clients. That is the extent to which CPNs were more positive than their clients about change exceeded the extent to which social workers were more positive than their clients.

These data, it should be emphasized, do not mean the clients were, overall, negative about change. Indeed, they generally (though not always) indicated some degree of positive change. However, in relation to social problems, they were less positive than the workers (and the CPNs in particular). This was also the case with CPNs for mental health problems. Furthermore, the clients, it should be remembered, were more uncertain in relation to mental health problems. However the implications are generally clear: viewed from the clients' standpoint, in relation to brief and extended work, and with both social and mental health problems, CPNs appear overconfident about the degree of change achieved. Social workers, on the other hand, underestimate, from the client's standpoint, the degree of positive mental health change although they too (albeit considerably less than CPNs) are more optimistic than clients about social problem change. The picture, however, may be rather better with extended work with emotional and relationship problems than it appears. Frequently, as shown earlier, social work clients defined as depression problems defined by the social worker as emotional. It may be that some of the 'negative gaps' between social workers and clients with emotional and relationship problems would be reduced if related to neurotic problems.

Conclusion

This chapter has examined issues relating to communication (or its likely effect) and client involvement in the process of intervention. Three broad conclusions come from this:

1   That concordance or agreement was generally greater with extended than with brief intervention;
2   That, again in general, social workers fare rather better than CPNs over a range of measures;
3   That clients are prepared, in a considerable minority of cases, to accept some responsibility for their problems, and generally see themselves as taking a large proportion of responsibility for managing their problems.

The data are however complex, and do not always point in the directions indicated here. Although, therefore, there tended to be greater concordance and agreement with extended intervention, more brief than extended clients agreed with the worker over primary problem and concordance was greater with brief than extended mental health problems. However, clients receiving extended intervention were more accurately aware of the workers' views of both mental health and social problems, as well as problems tackled. They agreed with the worker more frequently on the most effective activity, and showed, overall, a greater degree of satisfaction. Although there are exceptions, therefore, these data are consistent with a view that lengthier intervention offers greater opportunity for clarification and mutually agreed definitions of problems and work undertaken. However, it would be a mistake to be complacent about this. Such agreement does not follow automatically from extended intervention. There were considerable minorities and at times majorities of cases of discordance and disagreement between client and worker.

Although social workers generally fared better than CPNs over a wide range of measures, there were exceptions. The global measure of satisfaction showed social work clients tending to be more satisfied than CPN clients. This global rating is consistent with much, though not all, of the other measures. Those examining concordance or agreement reveal CPNs to fare better with primary problems (extended intervention), mental health problems (although this was reversed when worker defined emotional problems were included), and brief CPN clients were more accurate than social work clients in identifying workers' views of mental health problems. Concordance or agreement between social worker and client was higher than between CPN and client with primary problems (brief work) and social problems (brief and extended work). Social work clients were more accurately aware of workers' views and activities undertaken (brief and extended work). Other factors indicate deficiencies in CPN work not evident purely from measures of satisfaction. Over half the CPN clients, wanted some additional or alternative work (activities) undertaken. A noticeable deficiency was in psychodynamic work, interesting in view of the relatively low proportion of CPN cases receiving psychodynamic work identified in Chapter 5. Social workers undertaking extended intervention were, according to their clients, more actively involved in defining problems, planning and carrying out intervention. Finally, CPNs' clients were consistently and markedly more negative than the CPNs themselves in relation to the index of change. This 'negative gap' was consistently greater than that between social workers and their clients, who were generally more positive than the social workers themselves about mental health problems. The clients considered themselves to take a major responsibility in relation to their problems. Thus a considerable minority felt they had some responsibility for their problems in the first place. They also played, as far as they were concerned, the major role in defining problems, planning and carrying out work in relation to these problems, although social workers also played a greater role than CPNs. Finally, they perceived the focus to be very much on the client themselves, a focus with which, on the whole, they approved.

The picture of client worker interaction, therefore, is complex but throws up some interesting trends. Overall they suggest social work client agreement is greater than CPN client agreement and that social work clients are more aware of workers' problem definitions and activities (suggesting clearer communication). Other factors — particularly deficiencies in activities undertaken — are interesting in view of the smaller range of CPN activities identified in Chapter 5. Indeed, client perception of CPNs' involvement in the process of defining, planning and carrying out tasks suggests a curious *lack* of involvement by CPNs. It is as if CPNs were there, perhaps providing support, but not positively involved in problem resolution. This can be examined in greater depth through clients' accounts of intervention, which we shall turn to in the next chapter.

Note

1 Marital: social work 6 out of 6; CPN 0 out of 1; joint 2 out of 4. Social relations/isolation: social work 6 out of 7; CPN 3 out of 8; joint 2 out of 9.

Chapter 8

Client Perceptions: Brief Intervention

The analysis of interpersonal skills may be taken further by the examination of qualitative information gained from the client interviews. This has the advantage of allowing the clients to describe their experience of intervention and hence provide a complement to the more quantitative information. The central concern remains the analysis of professional skills and the replies of clients were subject to content analysis examining them through the framework of the skills identified in Chapter 6. Clients interviewed were asked a number of questions

1 On the whole, how satisfied were you with the service you received? They were given five alternatives ranging from very satisfied to very dissatisfied.

2 On the basis of their response they were asked the open ended question: what was it about the service you received that made you satisfied (or dissatisfied or neither satisfied nor dissatisfied)? At the end of this response they were asked: were there any other aspects of the service about which you felt satisfied (or dissatisfied or neither satisfied nor dissatisfied)?

3 If they felt satisfied, they were then asked: are there any aspects of the service about which you felt dissatisfied? If they felt dissatisfied the reverse question was asked.

4 Finally, they were asked: what difference, if any, would it have been made if the social worker/CPN had not been involved?

Three basic methods were used to identify skills from the clients' accounts. First there were direct statements of the skills which were used, for example where the worker was listening or understanding and empathic, these would be stated directly.

Table 8.1 Brief Intervention: Skills identified by clients

Relationship	Social Work	CPN	Joint
Care/commitment	6	4	6
Individualizing	1	—	1
Support	1	—	—
Empathy/understanding	6	—	5
Listening	10	6	7
Acceptance	6	2	3
Authentic — Genuine	2	—	—
Expert			
Increasing self understanding	1	1	—
Confronting	1	—	—
Clarifying	—	—	—
Release of feelings	—	—	2
Analytic processes	—	—	—
Advice	5	2	5
Information	1	2	1
Knowledge	3	—	3
TOTAL: Relationships	32 (2.5)	12 (0.9)	22 (1.7)
TOTAL: Expert	11 (0.8)	5 (0.4)	11 (0.8)
TOTAL OVERALL:	43 (3.3)	17 (1.3)	33 (2.5)

(Figures in brackets are the average number of relevant skills per case)

The way she was listening and the things she was saying in return.

or

I felt she was a really understanding woman — she really felt for me

Second, there were statements which described a skill without, however, stating it directly. For example in one case support was described:

She helped me negotiate a really bad period. She buoyed me up. . . .
I felt I had somebody other than my wife and children I could turn to.

Third, there were composite statements where more than one skill was described, as in one case where support, understanding and caring were cited:

I found [worker] very supportive, very understanding. She made me feel as though I was important to her outside the situation I was in.
I think it was as if she was a friend without being one.

Results in Table 8.1 show interesting and dramatic differences between occupations. There is a definite pecking order: social work clients identified more skills than joint clients and markedly more than CPN clients. Both social work and joint clients identified twice as many expert skills as CPN clients, and social work clients identified nearly three times the number of relationship qualities as CPN clients. It is also interesting that the relationship qualities identified by clients exceeded those of expert skills in all occupation groups by a ratio of 2:1 or more. Over the relatively brief period of this intervention, the ability to be human and concerned appears to have been most significant. Of the relationship qualities care and commitment and the ability to listen were most identified by clients from all groups. Interestingly, joint and social workers appear to have been markedly more able than CPNs to transmit empathy and understanding to their clients. Of expert skills, advice was most frequently cited. This is consistent with brief intervention: advice, whether practical or interpersonal, may be the most useful expert skill on offer in a relatively short time period. A profile of three skills: being able to listen, to empathize and understand and to give helpful advice appears most useful with brief intervention.

Social Work

Social work and joint clients were therefore aware of a wider display of skills than CPN clients. This trend — of CPNs performing least impressively — is broadly consistent with quantitative data analyzing client perspectives. Social work clients expressed recognition of relationship qualities in various ways. A number expressed recognition of *caring* or *commitment* by the worker. One stated it in terms of a variety of qualities cemented by concern:

> She was very helpful and sympathetic. I was feeling really down about my wife leaving and I needed to talk it through with someone who was not involved. She really seemed concerned. I didn't really expect that from a stranger.

Other clients stated similarly 'she was just very kind and helpful' or 'she was more or less comforting and seemed kind and caring'. Others saw evidence of commitment in the speed of response to the referral, particularly if no prior appointment was made: 'I was quite impressed by how quickly they dealt with me. I mean I didn't make an appointment or anything' or 'there's an immediate response.... I think myself that its a lot of reassurance if you're in trouble'. *Acceptance*, closely related to caring, was identified in various ways. One presented it in terms of the welcome she got:

> I felt very much at ease.... I felt quite welcome. I wasn't made to feel as if I was in an institution. It was a relaxed and comfortable atmosphere.

Others identified friendliness as a key aspect and a sense of belonging:

> I liked the welcome [worker] gave me. The feeling that I belonged. She was ever so friendly when I walked in. With a doctor you're in and out like a battery hen.

The most widely canvassed element of acceptance, however, was overt statements of not being judged. A consistent theme was vulnerability of client self esteem, both arising with their problems and their decision to seek help.

> She was really nice. I've been drinking a lot and I had to pluck up courage to go and see them. When I went there she didn't just discuss it and tell me to pull myself together, which I half expected her to do.

Another client (forcefully) advised to choose between wife and girlfriend after an affair, was aware of separation of self from acts when the worker said that, whatever he decided, he could come back again: 'she wasn't judging me or anything'. Indeed he had rather expected censure: 'she didn't have a go at me or anything which I thought she might'. Another client associated acceptance with an objective approach to intervention which made the whole process rather less traumatic.

Listening was the most widely identified social work skill. However, listening operated at different levels. One was passive listening — acting as a 'sounding board'. This was important for one client, the unfortunate subject of genetic attraction to her estranged father, whom she had met recently for the first time:

> It was just like someone to talk to. The sort of thing I could have said to my best friend, although I wouldn't have said this to my best friend.

Note here the importance of being separate from her social circle while possessing qualities normally associated with friends. Another client specifically referred to the worker as a 'sounding board', while another coupled such listening with confidentiality. For others listening was *active*, and was demonstrated by the worker's response, as with the worker who coupled listening with suggestions about voluntary work. Such listening could be sophisticated:

> she was a really good listener and adviser. She knew exactly when to let me talk and when to interrupt to give me advice.

The skill involved not simply giving appropriate advice, and hence showing 'real' listening, but knowing *how* to listen, which involves knowing when to be quiet and when to interrupt. Another client compared this real listening with their negative experience of others when 'it's as if people don't have the time or aren't interested'. This displays an element identified earlier: that the response was better than expected or previously experienced. Clients may judge workers in the context of their life experience. Thus another client referring positively to listening said:

> When I went there I didn't think I'd want to talk about it. I thought
> it would just be a waste of time.

A final element of listening was a combination of patience and giving time: 'they're professionals — you can be in a room with them and they give you time'. Another said:

> I think they should be quite receptive — be able to listen so you
> know they understand what you're talking about.

There are three elements here: the client has something to communicate, the worker hears *and* understands what is said, and the client knows they have understood.

Understanding is the aspect of *empathy* most evident. One client explicitly used a term reminiscent of the social work and nursing literature, when they said they should 'listen to you carefully and put themselves in your shoes'. Being understood was not just important in itself, but for its cathartic effect:

> I just felt better telling her. She seemed to understand what I was
> telling her.... If you talk to just anyone they don't really under-
> stand. But she knew about this sort of thing — they're trained really
> — and you need that to deal with these situations.

An additional element, knowledge and training, was emphasized. Understanding was not something just anyone could provide. However, another client identified it as a natural human quality:

> You can feel it with some people — they can make you feel at ease.
> Other people don't — just go up to see my doctor and you'll see
> what I mean.

One client linked understanding with sympathy appropriate to the problem's gravity: 'if you lose your husband that's more distressing than getting your money stolen or whatever'. However, another saw the importance of some distancing, 'to stand back' and 'to have that authoritative air'. Underlying understanding, for one client, was respect: the worker

> was very understanding and basically she took me quite seriously .... Most of all they should take what they [clients] say as gospel [although] I suppose they need to look out for when someone is hiding something.

Other qualities were less frequently cited. *Genuineness* was evident in one case in the worker's 'real' qualities, concern and interest:

> he was such a friendly person, he was someone you could trust, someone who didn't impose himself on you. He was someone you could talk to.

Another related it to honesty and sincerity, feeling she could 'trust what she's saying and what she's doing. She's pretty honest with you really ... very genuine.' Another spoke of *support* involving being treated seriously and objectively: 'he was more of a support — it was nice to blurt everything out.... I didn't sit there and feel stupid.' *Individualizing* was expressed by one client as 'the aim is on you yourself ... they can provide the situation where you can help yourself.'

The most frequently identified expert skill was *advice*. One client expressed this not in terms of goals but means of achieving them, speaking of 'pointers. How to get on your own feet. She suggested how I might be able to manage my life a bit more effectively'. Another likewise said 'they suggested ways I could try and deal with this [anxiety] which were really helpful'. Advice could be seen as preferred but not binding alternatives (non-directive): 'he gave me his opinion, but left the decision to me, whereas my mum tries to direct me — you've got to do this or do that'. Advice did not have to be softly delivered to be appreciated:

> The advice she gave me was rather blunt really, though thinking about it now it was the best advice perhaps ... she actually suggested to me to keep it [genetic attraction] to myself and if necessary to continue to see her.... I wish I'd taken her advice because I did [tell someone] and I regret it.

Closely associated for some clients was the importance of *knowledge*. One client was surprised by their expertise. She was

> better than I expected. She knew much more than I thought. Its difficult to say exactly what. She seemed to know about handling emotions and things.

Another recognized the importance of training to 'know about this sort of thing', while another identified it through appropriate scepticism: 'they're knowledgeable ... you can't fool them for a minute'. Information was provided for one client through 'a few suggestions about voluntary work'. One client felt the worker had *increased self understanding*. This is interesting because this might generally be considered a longer term process. Nonetheless it had a great impact on the client, who considered it 'amazing':

> She was very perceptive. She seemed able to draw things out of me so that I became aware of things that I hadn't really thought of before. Amazing really ... it really helped to clear my mind.

Confronting, finally, occurred with one client, a man who was having an affair was urged to decide between his wife and lover:

> she said I had better get my act together. It did make me stand up a bit. I couldn't play one off against the other. I'd have to decide which one I was going to stay with.

Joint Work

Interpersonal skills were identified less frequently by clients subject to joint work. This is interesting, for it further questions an assumption about joint work: that workers bringing skills specific to their discipline would, when combined, provide clients with a better service. Indeed, this is consistent with the examination of both practice and theory foundations of social work and nursing. The latter appear, with the exception of their specialist mental health diagnostic training, to offer little additional to the former.

Like social work clients, joint clients perceived *commitment* in the speed of response to the referral. One who had expected to be 'there all day ... wasn't kept waiting at all' and another commented that 'it was quick — I didn't have to wait a day or so'. Again in some cases it was viewed in terms of previous experience:

> when I see my [district] social worker I usually have to wait quite a while — once I had to wait about an hour.

The commitment displayed by speedy responses could be significant to desperate clients: 'I was in a bit of a state at the time and I needed to see someone quickly.' Concern could be expressed in the energy with which clients were helped:

> They seemed genuinely concerned.... They put themselves out to contact people who could sort out the problems I had.

Concern was displayed not simply by 'doing things' for clients but was shown in the way workers presented themselves: 'the way you're dealt with on the phone; you're not dealt with clinical precision, like a name or number'.

Listening was the skill most frequently identified by joint workers' clients. Like social work clients some clients expressed it simply in the opportunity to talk: 'they actually sat back and let me talk'. Others coupled listening with other qualities: acceptance or being taken seriously:

> their approach — the way they listened and made me talk. They didn't tell you 'for God's sake drop it or whatever'. They approached the matter as I thought it should be approached.

Another said 'they really listened and took me seriously. I didn't get any help at all from my husband — he just shouts at me'. Again, worker qualities were measured against previous experience. Being given time was important: 'they've got time. It seems when you see doctors they're so busy. You want somebody to listen to you'. However one difference from social work clients was evident: when two workers are involved, it may be important for both to listen:

> sometimes you are worried about one not listening, but they both got involved. Like from time to time each of them would make a comment which made it obvious they were taking notice.

Where this didn't occur it could be problematic:

> the social worker didn't say much — she listened, and was interested. The other wouldn't let you talk — she was more interested in what she thought and had to say.

This criticism reveals some key elements: being attentive to what the client says, not interrupting at inappropriate times and letting the client set the agenda.

Empathy or understanding could mean being treated seriously:

> the first thing is understanding. That you're not some kind of freak or you're not just doing it to be clever. They do have the knowledge and the professional status — they are aware of what you're going through.

This man, anxious and depressed by work pressures, linked the ability to understand with knowledge and professional status. Others stressed ordinariness as well as knowledge: 'it's just down to earth people who seem to understand'. For others understanding involved a wide appreciation of the client's position: 'they showed they completely grasped the situaton and understood it'. While another emphasized the importance of an immediate sense of understanding: 'you get that feeling right from when you walk in . . . really important when you're upset or anything'. Another client stressed personal experience for empathy, perhaps taking it too far:

> I don't think anybody can understand what its like unless they've had a nervous breakdown. I think they should all have nervous break-downs — doctors do, I know — lots of them.

Other qualities identified included *acceptance* which could involve being non-censorious, favourably contrasted with others' judgmental attitude: 'they had no high and mighty attitude — they didn't say the situation was all my fault like most people do'. Acceptance could contribute to the provision of advice acceptable to the client. One man estranged from his wife said 'without telling me I'd done the wrong thing they told me I should stop fighting it and concentrate more on myself'.

Advice, as with social work, was the most frequently identified expert skill, often linked with *knowledge*: 'I feel they've got to be really qualified to help.... I want to be given advice based on knowledge'. Another client commented:

> they're very knowledgeable — on the one hand they can settle you down — then they talk to you and tell you simple straightforward things at first and then go into more detail which is helpful.

Here the process of advice giving is significant: the calming effect followed by simple advice and then more detail — going at the client's pace. For another client the advice was welcome because it was consistent with their views: 'I had a pretty good idea of what was wrong, but its really helpful to have it confirmed by others who know what they're talking about'. Another client placed advice in the context of experiences elsewhere: 'they explained things to you more than doctors do'. One woman considered it a bonus to have two workers:

> I think it was better that there were two rather than one person. They both were able to make suggestions and you felt they might come up with more suggestions.

Release of feelings was a further element identified by clients:

> they let me calm myself down. I was very angry.... They let me talk. I told them more or less everything. By the time I finished I'd got rid of a lot of pent up feelings.

Another said 'I needed to talk to someone — I was really pouring it out — but they didn't seem to mind'. Both cases indicate a spontaneous release of feelings waiting to burst out. The skills involved here, although important, are perhaps less than skills required at time to 'unlock' feelings which may be denied (e.g. unresolved grief reaction long after bereavement).

CPNs

CPN clients identified considerably fewer skills than either joint or social work clients. *Caring* or *commitment* were considered important by some clients, and as previously noted, may be considered in the light of experiences elsewhere:

> from my eyes, doctors don't really care. They just show you in and push you out. I think [the CPN] shows an interest in you and I have actually found that caring.

Others saw an element of professionalism in caring 'professionalism tempered by compassion' but 'they must have a certain amount of compassion because if you're too detached you lose this'. Other clients, as noted earlier, identified commitment through the speed of response to referral, of great importance to those who felt desperate, and a preparedness actually to visit the client rather than ask them to the Centre. One client commented that 'if you're feeling that desperate they do come out' although 'they might not help very much'. Clearly here the client was separating the act of caring from the actual helpfulness of the CPN. *Listening* was the most frequently cited skill. Like other clients, they identified different levels. There were those, like the woman with alcohol problems, who simply needed to talk:

> it helps to talk. Simply — it helps to talk. . . . I've had a lot down my throat and I felt better when I spoke to her.

Others regarded listening as more active: hence the CPN 'listened and then she went outside and tried to find some way to help me out'. Others compared the response with other people:

> There's one or two people down this way. They don't listen to you, they laugh at you. This young man sat and listened. He was charming.

However, there could be reservations: listening on its own may not be enough.

Table 8.2 *Brief Intervention: Criticisms related to skills*

	Social Work	CPN	Joint
Relationship	4	6	6
Expert	5	13	5
TOTAL	9	19	11

> they only listened and did nothing. It's difficult to say really — they just came here, listened and then they went ... they didn't do a lot to resolve the problem.

Acceptance was demonstrated for one client by the respect they received:

> his general manner was good. He wasn't abrupt. He was polite. He knew the situation and he treated me in a respectful way.

For another it was being non-censorious, comparing the CPN with others 'you get so much criticism by some others. They shouldn't criticize, they should just talk. It just brings you down'.

Expert skills were rarely identified. *Advice* and *information* predominated. One client discussed their drink problem with a CPN:

> he was telling me not the good side of it but the bad side of it.... I knew drink would damage you but he did it in more detail.

Another considered suggestions helpful because they were a 'relevant response' to their problems, while merely informing a client about a day centre indicated to them that the CPN 'tried to find some way to help us out'. Another client felt the CPN had *increased* his *self understanding* (person — situation reflection).

> It made me look at areas that I didn't actually think about. Even when I went there just once they began to pinpoint areas which I hadn't really seen before myself.

Criticisms of Workers

While social work clients identified the most skills and CPN clients the least skills, negative comments about skills were made most frequently by CPN clients. This accentuated the disparity between the occupations. On relationship qualities two social work clients felt they were not genuinely interested (i.e. *did not care*). One client, with a 12.30 appointment was asked to wait an hour:

I didn't think she was very interested in me ... if it was arranged I shouldn't have had to wait that hour. She should put her lunch back.

Another considered it 'dubious' they could be interested 'after a number of years at the job'. One client cited *lack of support* ('emotional and moral') 'I didn't ask her specifically for this — I expected she would identify this — for her to offer that to me'. Another said 'when I saw her she was a bit rude actually ... she came at me like a ton of bricks'. *Lack of advice* where it was expected could be a problem 'even though I wasn't necessarily looking for any answers, she didn't make any suggestions'. When advice came it was not considered good advice:

she also suggested working abroad — going to a kibbutz — but I thought it was rather daft. It's a bit like running out on the situation.

Another suggested they 'needed more time with her' and 'she didn't give me enough suggestions'. One client felt the worker *failed to increase understanding* of herself or her situation. She was expected to tell the worker her problems, and was listened to, but

it was a bit like 'bare your soul' with no gain you know? I had really hoped that she'd be able to sort of unravel my thoughts.

Joint workers were also subject to criticism. One complained of a *lack of concern*, a kind of flatness betokening disinterest:

they were neither excited nor worried by me going. They weren't going to think about me after I left. They weren't horrible to me or anything but also I didn't think it mattered very much to them.

This was expressed also by a woman who felt 'they weren't very sympathetic' about her financial difficulties. Another complained the workers were intolerant: he found it offputting that they looked at each other 'with a pained expression on their face as if to say "when is this guy going to go?"' Two clients felt patronized by the workers: one complaining they were 'talking down to me as if I was a child and didn't understand this that and the other'. The other felt:

it was like she was scoring points — she said she was a single parent and she had to manage — and I ended up asking her what I should do. I felt a bit inadequate really.

Another client, unemployed with serious financial difficulties, complained of a *complete lack of understanding* — an inability to tune in to the extent of the problem.

They didn't seem to realize my difficulties. All they said was that we all have financial problems, like mortgages ... but it's not the same when you don't get much money. How are you going to save when you're on Social Security?

Lack of advice could be a problem. One case indicated a failure to 'tune in' properly: a woman living in a deprived area, who wanted a move and had hoped for a letter of support to the housing department, was told she had 'done the home up and I should go and see people more'. Another hoping for advice 'was left to follow my own devices with no practical advice whatsoever', while one man complained they only listened: 'they let me talk a bit. They didn't give me any advice. At the end I thought "so what".'

One client felt he had not been assessed properly because he needed further help; he did not get 'to go there a number of times and gradually get rid of the problem'. A final general complaint of *no skill* was made:

the whole thing came across as immature amateurs trying hard to do a professional job and doing it badly. I don't feel they had any qualifications whatsoever.

The CPNs were subject to most criticisms. Five clients referred to a *lack of commitment or concern* by the CPN, or not being taken seriously. One complained

they just seemed to go through the motions. There's nothing they did to help me.... I think they classified me as 'she's not really got problems'.... There's nothing worse when you're crying your eyes out than for someone to sit there and look at you.

Another client complained that the CPN 'didn't seem very interested at all' and that there 'wasn't enough time to talk about why I was there'. A further client felt their problems were not taken seriously. The CPN said of their severe financial problems 'you seem to have it under control', additionally 'she seemed to take no notice of what I said about the children'. One client felt a sense of detachment:

I found [CPN] a little too detached. She didn't really seem warm. I just felt as if she wasn't particularly interested and she was just paid to listen.

Another complained of 'their whole attitude — they seemed rather self centred'. He said, 'it was left to me to do all the talking and give all the answers — I felt like "what am I doing here?"' One client complained of *lack of support*: 'they weren't very supportive. Although they let me talk there wasn't much support behind it'.

Criticism of expert skills was more extensive. Bad or non-existent advice was a particular problem. One woman who had lost her baby felt advice failed to account for her circumstances:

> their advice wasn't up to much. I could understand if they said get over it if I hadn't got a job — but when I have to go to work ten hours a night and then come back to run a house — it was too much.

A woman advised to go to a MIND day centre said she 'didn't really want to spend Sunday with a load of depressed people'. Four people complained of a lack of advice where it was expected, for example: 'I felt they sat there just listening and that was it — goodbye. They didn't really give a lot of advice' or 'they didn't give me any advice at all'. Another woman received advice — to go to an alcohol unit — but did not like it:

> I just thought no way am I going to be lectured by someone — like having to stand up while other people are sitting around and listening to your problems.

Clients also complained about the ability to analyze and identify problems. One said the CPN 'didn't really ask me anything which might have helped me understand what was going on'. Another client felt the CPN focused on the wrong problem, working to a different agenda:

> he seemed mainly concerned with my drink problem, but I hadn't come there for that. He wasn't interested in my housing problem or the rows I was having with my girlfriend.

Another client who wanted counselling said 'it was not on the level I wanted'. Others complained the CPN simply did nothing:

> I did feel rather like I was sitting there saying things while they just hummed and haad. They didn't actually help me to begin to resolve my problems or make any suggestions.

Other clients said 'they just come here, listen to what I had to say and then went' or 'I was doing all the talking and they didn't do anything'. Some CPN work was, therefore, masterly (or not so masterly) inactivity.

The Impact of Intervention

There is, then, a clear and consistent pattern. Clients of social workers were more positive and less negative about skills than either joint workers or CPNs, the latter clearly faring the worst. However, skills relate primarily to

Table 8.3 Brief Intervention: Impact of worker involvement

	Social Work	CPN	Joint	Total
Worsened situation	—	—	1	1
No difference	4	6	6	16
Temporary support only	3	1	2	6
Facilitated help from others	—	2	3	5
Problems would have remained/ worsened	4	3	—	7
Catalyst (helping clients to change their circumstances)	2	1	1	4

process of intervention rather than outcome. In relation to the latter, clients were asked: What difference, if any, would it have made if the social worker and/or CPN had not been involved?

Client replies were grouped according to their responses, shown in table 8.3. For seventeen clients (44 per cent) intervention made no difference or worsened their situations, while others felt some help was given. As with other measures, CPN results were least positive. However the pattern of response varied between client groups. In particular CPN and joint clients felt workers had facilitated help from others where social work clients did not, while no CPN clients felt the problems would have remained or worsened, though a number of social work and joint clients did.

The client responses in come cases graphically illustrate these data. Only one (CPN) client felt the worker actually worsened the situation, a woman with an unresolved grief reaction to her child's cot death:

> there was nothing really that they did that helped me. In fact I felt worse after they'd been ... they just seemed to say its about time I got over it. I was really exhausted.... I felt more depressed when they left.

Others felt it made no difference, though for various reasons. For some it meant the worker had done nothing, and the client was quite dismissive: 'it used up some of my valuable time' or 'I had to go away and cope with it myself' or 'they didn't actually do anything'. Others were not critical, but felt that help would be better provided elsewhere, or accepted that little could be achieved to help them: one man was looking for medical treatment, another considered their doctor to be their main help, while another still considered the referral itself was 'all a big mistake and should have gone elsewhere'. One client said it made no difference, but, having been referred on, 'I hope when I see someone else, something will come out of it'.

Others actually regarded the gatekeeping providing access to other professionals or resources positively (facilitating help from others).

For example, one client said

> they were really practical. They got on to housing and social security and tried to sort it out. Someone's coming round to see me about it.

Another felt empowered in their relationship with their doctor because they were being given advice, on tablets they were prescribed by their doctor, information of which they were previously unaware, and a further client felt helped by referral to a day centre. Where clients suggested the problem would have remained or got worse, the intervention, though brief, made a considerable difference. One client with difficulties with their partner said

> if I hadn't gone I would have just sat and stewed and it would have taken a lot longer to get over it. I mean you've got your parents to talk to, but they're subjective.

Another said

> I think it would have made a hell of a lot of difference.... I probably would have got worse — I really was in some state.

The worker, finally, could act as a catalyst for change. One client, for example, said

> oh a big difference. I felt I was looking at things through a haze beforehand. Now although I still feel pretty bad I see things a lot more clearly.

Another said

> they did help me a load, but you've got to want to get on your feet yourself. They can't do it themselves. When I left there I certainly wanted to resolve things.

Comments

A number of interesting elements arise from these clients' responses. The first is that although intervention was brief the analysis of client responses shows an awareness of a variety of skills. Of these skills it is the relationship qualities rather than expert skills which predominate, although the latter do appear. This suggests, first, that clients themselves, even those receiving brief intervention, are capable of telling us important elements of practice. Viewed through the framework of skills considered important in the literature, we get a clear picture of the skills experienced by the clients. It also suggests that, for many of these clients, the experience of being taken seriously and related to with genuine human concern was very important. Third, this balance between relationship qualities and expert skills may occur primarily with brief intervention: that when contact is short it is possible to demonstrate quickly important human qualities, but less easy to develop and display some of the expert skills. However, two further points may be made. As a community mental health setting, the agency may have attracted more emotional problems relative to practical problems than perhaps some other settings, such as Area Social Service teams. For people undergoing distress and crisis the demonstration of warmth may provide the most immediate impact. Second, some expert skills, particularly relating to areas such as clarifying or increasing self understanding may actually be difficult for clients to express clearly — hence reducing the frequency of their presence in client responses.

A further theme identifiable from time to time is one which will surprise few researchers: that there is evidence that clients make judgments in the context of their experiences elsewhere. Judgments about workers can arise through direct comparison with other people. Some of the comments about other experiences are very disparaging: the doctors who give them little time and less interest; relatives or friends who are simply not concerned with their problems; the husband who, worse still, shouts at the woman who tries to discuss her problems with him, and so on. In such a context, workers' preparedness simply to listen or show concern is likely to be experienced very positively, even when intervention is brief. Of course that is not to deny that some of the relationship qualities practised by these professionals may involve high levels of skill — for example reaching for feeling in the process of displaying empathy. However, it is also noticeable that there are times when caring and listening were simply not enough. In particular this was the case when advice was being sought and it was either considered inadequate or non-existent, a complaint made by a number of clients. This emphasizes the point made at the outset: that with brief intervention a triad of skills are most important to clients — being able to listen, to empathize and understand, and to give helpful advice.

The picture, though, is not entirely rosy. It is noticeable that a high proportion (44 per cent) of clients felt intervention had made no difference or worsened the situation. Of course only one felt intervention had actually worsened things, but many who felt it made no difference appeared to feel rather let down. This may well be linked particularly with complaints about lack of advice. However, there are considerable variations between professional groups, although the variations point broadly in one direction: social work clients identified more skills, made fewer criticisms about misused or unused skills and less frequently suggested their intervention made no difference than either CPN or joint clients. CPNs, on the other hand, fared worst in all three respects, and by noticeable margins. Indeed over half of these CPN clients suggested they made no difference or worsened the situation. It would appear, that, with brief intervention anyway, the clients' experience varied greatly depending upon the group which saw them. Furthermore, there is also an indication that, again from the clients' experience, joint work does *not* lead to a better service. Indeed the involvement of two people might add extra potential strains, as suggested by the client who emphasized the importance of involvement by both professionals. While of course these are the responses of only a sample of all clients, the evidence is consistent with the greater skills manifested by social workers discussed previously in the book. However, matters may differ with extended intervention and it is to this we shall now turn.

Chapter 9

Client Perceptions:
Extended Intervention

While marked differences are evident from brief intervention, it does not follow that these will occur with extended intervention. Stuart Rees (1974) has discussed how particular problems may arise — especially in client-worker perceptions — when intervention is so brief that it involves no more than contact. Furthermore, earlier chapters have suggested marked differences between brief and extended intervention in what CPNs and social workers actually do. The separate examination of extended intervention may well, therefore repay analysis. Table 9.1 shows the skills identified by clients. A number of factors are immediately apparent. First, clients identified a greater average number of skills per case than with brief intervention, by a factor of 1.4:1 for social workers and 2.1:1 for CPNs. This was fairly consistent. For both CPNs and social workers, and across both relationship qualities and expert skills, extended clients identified, on average, more skills than brief clients. This is interesting because it suggests that longer term intervention allowed the workers to display, or at least clients appreciate, more skills, However, we must remember that more extended intervention gives client and worker greater opportunity to build a relationship, which may in turn either help the client to view the worker more positively or alternatively induce a sense of obligation which makes them reluctant to criticize the worker. However, this might be expected to occur primarily in global statements of satisfaction: more detailed analysis may reveal greater details of strengths and weaknesses. Furthermore, it may be that, where stated in more detail, positive comments (given a relationship was built) would relate, in these circumstances, to the qualities of the worker. However there was an increase both in relationship *and* expert skills identified with extended intervention. It seems reasonable to suppose, therefore, that these data reflect a genuine difference in the skills experienced by clients receiving extended compared with brief intervention.

The other major point is that social workers' clients again experienced a greater number of skills than CPN clients. Furthermore the gap, in terms of

Table 9.1   Extended Intervention: Skills identified by clients

Relationship	Social Work	CPN
Care — commitment	12	10
Individualizing	3	1
Support	10	5
Empathy/understanding	13	6
Listening	13	5
Acceptance	6	5
Authentic — genuine	—	1
Expert		
Increasing self understanding	4	2
Clarifying	1	—
Release feelings	5	—
Analytic processes	6	2
Advice	8	7
Information	6	—
Knowledge	—	—
Encouraging — enabling	—	1
TOTAL: Relationship	57 (3.0)	39 (2.1)
TOTAL: Expert	30 (1.6)	13 (0.7)
OVERALL TOTAL	87 (4.6)	52 (2.7)

(Figures in brackets represent the average number of skills per case)

ratios, is wider with expert skills (2.3:1) than relationship qualities (1.5:1), leaving an overall ratio of 1.7:1. The pattern of skills is rather different for CPNs and social workers. Listening, care and commitment and advice stand out for CPNs, similar to the overall picture for brief intervention. However, while listening, empathy and understanding and care and commitment stand out as social worker relationship qualities, information, analytic processes and release of feelings as well as advice are noticeable as expert skills. There is, then, a wider range of expert skills found helpful by extended social work clients than clients receiving brief intervention. Of course, these comments are made in the light of frequently different purposes of brief compared with extended intervention, the former involved frequently with assessment, referral and short term support, the latter with longer term psychosocial help.

Social Work

These results, then, indicate again that social work clients experienced intervention markedly differently, as a group, from CPN clients. As with brief intervention these clients experience relationship qualities in various ways. *Caring or commitment* was identified by nearly two-thirds of the clients interviewed. One middle-aged woman whose husband had left her emphasized its importance:

> She couldn't have been a more caring person. I don't know exactly how she showed it — she kept making me feel I was a worthwhile person, that I had a lot to live for and a lot to give.

Caring for this woman was a mysterious process, but she recognized respect and lifting her self esteem as key aspects. For others it took some burden of responsibility off their shoulders: 'I felt a great sense of relief. I felt I'd been able to hand over the reins ... someone on the end of the phone who would care'. This can involve support, and suggests a close relationship between caring and support in practice. For others it maintained involvement: 'if I'd been met by a cold, clinical unresponsive lot I probably wouldn't have come back'. A further dimension was the relationship one client made between trust and caring: 'you need to have trust in somebody, that's the important thing ... if you trust somebody you can confide in them and they won't repeat what you've told them'. Confidentiality, then was for this client an aspect of caring. For extended clients commitment was demonstrated by the responsiveness of workers: 'the fact that I didn't have to wait long to see someone and the fact that when I did I didn't have to wait long to see them again. They were responsive and prompt'. Others also emphasized commitment demonstrated not just at the beginning but throughout the intervention as with one woman who could 'pick up the phone' and the worker would respond and another whose worker was prepared to come outside office hours.

> Good Friday she came to see me. Not many people work on Good Friday. I felt as though I could turn to her no matter when I needed her and she'd come quickly.

Another saw the worker's commitment in the thoroughness of her preparation: 'she had obviously taken the trouble to find out facts I needed to know before I went ... she was really well prepared ... she was professional'. Overall caring and commitment differed in one respect with extended compared with brief intervention. Clients tended to speak of it as a process where it was continually re-demonstrated, whereas with brief intervention it was demonstrated on the whole as an immediate once off process.

Support was an element emphasized by many clients. One woman felt the very presence of the social worker made her feel more secure: 'the moment I walked through the door I felt safe. I felt this is it. I've got the help I need'. Others did not have this touching faith, and required some demonstration of support. One client described this as something which 'made me feel less isolated' and another said:

> it gave me a lift just to see her. She always encouraged me when I felt things got difficult — like I didn't feel up to doing anything she got me out and going down the shops.

Another woman, reacting adversely to news that she was sterile, emphasized that social work support gave her confidence:

> she helped give me confidence to make the way I felt clearer to him [husband]. At the time my confidence had been completely shattered — it had since my mum died and now everything seemed to close in on me.

One client commented on the support gained from a combination of individual and group work: 'it's helpful to know there are other people who are suffering — you don't feel so alone'.

As with brief intervention, the ability to *empathize* with or understand the client was significant. One man, wrongly accused of stealing at work and depressed said, 'I felt she was a really understanding woman — she really felt for me. I could see she was on my side'. Being on his side was clearly important for this innocent man. Another client described empathy well — somewhere between over-involvement in client problems and dismissiveness:

> I was really down in the dumps at one time, and she seemed to understand what I felt — really well. It wasn't 'pull yourself together' or 'oh dear I'm sorry'. It seemed to be somewhere in between.

Another, who had experience of counselling, put it equally well: 'I got a dispassionate view. It's the difference between empathy and sympathy. I didn't want someone to dive in and drown with me'. Others, reminiscent of brief clients' comments, indicated judgment was made based on past experience. One woman compared the workers' empathy with her husband: 'he was stubborn. I'd explain them [problems] to him and he'd say "that's not right — it's something else". She could accept what I said as straight'. Another client emphasized others' insensitivity:

> trouble is you talk to other people and they don't know how to read you — she did.

Listening, a skill closely related to empathy, was also valued by some clients. Listening could be linked to a helping input such as advice:

> she helped me to pull through. It wasn't practical things like money, it was more emotional like. She gave me good advice and she really listened well.

For others a display of interest was sufficient to indicate listening.

> A bit like an agony aunt sort of effect — like Clare Raynor. Everybody needs somebody to talk to.... She really listened and seemed interested.

Another commented that 'she gives me a helluva lot of time — I mean some of them say "yeah, yeah, yeah" — they're not listening but I felt she was listening', while one woman mentioned 'the way she was listening and things she was saying in return'. Some saw listening requiring skills out of the ordinary, but, in one case difficult to identify:

> I think it was because somebody was prepared to listen.... I think perhaps she might have a special ability — I mean she's a trained social worker.

However, others were less aware of any special skills. For them listening was an essentially human ability, operating in one case like a friend: 'I felt I could talk to her — open up to her.... I really felt comfortable with her. You felt it was a friend that was coming around'. The professional role required incorporation of the 'real' person: listening was allied to genuineness.

Acceptance was another positive dimension of social work intervention. One woman related it to being given time to recover (from the death of both parents):

> probably the fact that she was more experienced. Instead of telling me to pull myself together ... she gave me time. She said it wouldn't happen this week or next week but I'd get there in the end.

Other clients' responses indicate skills related in a way they felt difficult to distinguish from each other:

> the general support and caring that was given. Understanding as well. There was no telling you you were wrong, you shouldn't be doing this.

For this client, acceptance was linked closely to support, caring and under-standing. Comments on acceptance, like other qualities, could occur in the context of client expectations. This did not necessarily, as in the other cases, involve reference to previous experience, but could relate to expectations based on the imagined nature of the service. One client, a heavy drinker, had expected the worker to react negatively:

> I felt slightly self conscious when I went there ... [worker] didn't try to lecture me or anything, she just tried to make helpful sugges-tions. She never told me it was all my fault or anything like that.

Advice was the most frequently cited expert skill. In some cases it related primarily to emotional problems:

at that time I was very down. I was going deeper and deeper into a block — which she actually told me ... she gave me a lot of advice. I wouldn't have been able to get out of it without that.

Another client said likewise: 'it wasn't practical things like money, it was more emotional. She gave me good advice'. Others did identify more practical advice right down to the performance of tasks:

she put over to me ... to let other people do things for me.... The way she put it was let other people look after you for the moment. Even the basics of coming here [to stay at sister's] so I'd be eating properly.

Likewise a client, separated from her husband and with difficulty keeping up with her mortgage repayment, was considerably more impressed with advice from her social worker — to sell the house and buy one she could afford — than advice from her family. *Information* provision was generally mentioned by clients in the context of other skills. Information was given on the basis of knowledge of the distress suffered. One depressed woman said 'she certainly seemed to make things better — talking to me and explaining things to me'. Another depressed woman spoke similarly:

I was finding it difficult to go and meet neighbours and friends. She told me that this was not an unusual reaction and many people reacted like that.... I felt less strange for feeling that way.

Such information on the process of distress was reassuring for the client. Like advice, information could also be practical, as with the worker who went through welfare benefits before the client then went to make a benefit claim.

Release of feelings was of great importance to some clients. One woman, sexually abused in her adolescence by her father, had never been able to work through the feelings of anger she felt against him. She said but for the worker 'things would have dragged on. I needed to talk. I needed to bring things out in the open which I couldn't do before'. Others felt that contact with a worker gave them 'permission' to let out their feelings. One said:

it was a place where I'd talk to them, they'd talk to me and we'd try to deal with things — it was a place where I could express my feelings.

Another client referred to the way the release of feelings was connected with her ability to think more clearly: 'it made me think and I was able to let go of my feelings I couldn't elsewhere. I really wouldn't have been able to do this so quickly or easily elsewhere'.

Increasing self understanding was an important source of satisfaction for some clients. One woman, who periodically became depressed, and appeared to be constantly doing things for others said,

> she opened my eyes a lot about myself. The way I was trying to help other people. I was taken for a mug basically.

Another commented on the way the social worker made insightful observations about them, '[you] see your own problems more clearly through seeing yourself through other people'. One client extended this to include group and individual sessions, both of which 'actually made me think about who I am, what I think about things and why I react to them as I do'. Another woman whose husband had left her felt she had no strength to carry on. However,

> she made me see that my children would bear the pain and she made me see things I could manage on my own if I had to.

Analytic processes were identified primarily in terms of assessment and exploration. One woman, with both marital and child care difficulties saw the process of exploration expanding the possibilities available:

> she explored areas I hadn't thought of and could not have got from my friends and relatives ... it come up with what I wanted, even though I didn't know at the time what I wanted.

Another client spoke similarly of the workers' systematic approach: 'she was able to examine all the options — to decide whether I needed hospital or other alternatives to that'. Others comments included those that the worker had been able to 'broaden my horizons as far as job or career opportunities available to me' or the ability to identify 'more options than a doctor could offer'. The connection between assessment and possible change is interesting here: the process of exploration can make the client feel helped because of the identification of options which might be pursued.

CPNs

Care or *commitment* had a high profile in the relationship qualities mentioned by CPN clients. One explained its importance to people in distress:

> the way you are when you're really depressed it's very awkward because you can tell if somebody doesn't really care and isn't interested in you. You've got to be interested in someone to do a job like that.

A woman, suffering from anxiety and serious physical ill health connected sincerity and concern with the time the CPN spent with her: 'he was always prepared to fit round me for interviews' while another considered their CPN caring in simple practical tasks: 'she went around and did some shopping for me and other practical things'. As identified already, clients saw the speed of caring in simple practical tasks: 'she went around and did some shopping for me and other practical things'. As identified already, clients saw the speed of response to referral indicating commitment by CPNs: 'I was very bad early in the morning ... a nurse was here before midday'. For others it was the consistent availability of CPNs rather than the initial response which was significant: 'She was always there when you wanted her. Sometimes I couldn't manage. I was frightened. Nighttimes are worst'.

Listening, as with social work, was important. Some clients referred to CPNs as sounding boards: 'when you're, talking they don't interrupt ... they listen to what you're saying and let you carry on till you've finished'. Others were also recipients of passive listening, but they could be ambivalent about it:

> [CPN] was a good listener. He was really easy to talk to, but you can't often tell what he's thinking. They're all like that though — if you always told people what you thought of them you could make them worse.

Listening for one client involved broadmindedness, a preparedness not to impose views upon the clients. It implied taking seriously what they were saying. The CPN

> was able to listen. A lot of people don't want to listen. They have their own views ... they have to be open and broadminded.

Some clients related the ability to listen to the quality of patience, as with one woman, depressed following the birth of her baby, and with little support from her husband, who said,

> patience is important. She was prepared to sit there and listen to you as long as necessary rather than give the impression 'I've got to be going'.

The same point was made by another woman who compared it with the 'next please' mentality of the doctor's surgery, and believed it necessary because 'you need to have time to actually find out what's wrong'. *Empathy*, again, was discussed in terms of understanding. One woman seriously physically ill felt a desperate need to be taken seriously, but where other people were saying pull yourself together he was more understanding. He was prepared to suggest going back to the doctors if you are not satisfied.

Another client, again comparing with experiences elsewhere, considered the understanding 'made me feel more relaxed than I could in front of my family' while another contrasted it with bossiness, 'saying I've got to do this or do that'. For this client this would have been a waste of time: 'I'd have reacted strongly against someone telling me what to do'. Understanding seemed to involve space to make her own choices. One man described key elements of empathy:

empathy with people — that they can understand them and be in touch with the feelings the person's trying to describe or has been through. There would be nothing worse than saying they understood what you've been through and then go off on a completely different track.

Here empathy is not something passive. If the CPN went on to other issues, the client would feel a lack of empathy. Additionally, empathy is wide ranging: the CPN understands the client as far as they are in touch with the client's feelings.

Other qualities identified included *acceptance*. For one client this clearly involved separating his own value from his acts, an elderly man who felt depressed said 'she didn't lose her temper — I'd nod off in the middle of her talking, and she'd just wake me up.' A woman, set tasks to perform, week by week, was impressed by the CPN's failure to condemn her when she did not actually do them. Others recognized it in terms of the 'friendly manner' of the worker, indicating no judgment about them as people: 'she came more or less as a friend' or 'she had a friendly manner' which 'put me at my ease'. *Support* was also commented on by some clients. One woman graphically described its importance in relation to depression as

a crutch to lean on. You know when you're like it yourself you think there's no end. But they've seen people like you before and they know there's life after depression. They can see you're getting better when you're not really aware of it yourself.

Others related it to encouragement: a client began to feel stronger 'in myself' because the CPN 'helped me build up my life again and build up my confidence', while one man commented on the encouragement received coming off medication for anxiety. One client remarked on the *individualized* service, 'the individual attention which was what I was really looking for', while another commented the CPN was 'not like a person paid to do psychiatry' reflecting the genuineness, for him, of the worker.

As with all groups, brief and extended, *advice* was the most appreciated expert skill. Indeed it was quite predominant, reflecting the narrower range of CPN, compared with social work, skills identified by clients. One man, whose wife had left him, felt he had been unable to move forward before receiving the practical and interpersonal advice of the CPN. The CPN was

> able to give you advice on how to handle situations where you've got problems with other people ... he made constructive suggestions which they [his family] didn't, like getting a new flat or accepting that I couldn't see my kids.

Advice could also be about appropriate behaviour: one woman, who overdosed after her boyfriend left, said

> I had this complex — people were looking at me all the time. I wouldn't go out. I was going to give up my job and everything. But [she] gave me advice that this was silly and that I should go out and I was somehow able to take her up on it.

In both cases the advice was freeing the clients from the constraints of their own limited perspectives or misperceptions of the situation. For others advice was a step by step process to help recovery, as with the elderly depressed man to whom the CPN 'suggested different things' such as getting out of bed early, and various tasks around the home to keep him occupied. Other expert skills, such as *increasing self understanding* were limited. A woman whose boyfriend had recently left her commented that her CPN 'helped me realize what a berk I was, involved with him [and] ... helped me look to the future' while another said 'the CPN help[ed] me understand more about myself. Mostly work and my relationship with my parents. I'd never really thought about it before'. *Analytic processes*, as with social work were expressed in terms of questions designed to assess the client and his situation, for example the client who said he 'asked me a lot of questions, although I know this was to try and find out about me so he could see if he could help'. One client, considering the CPN *knowledgeable*, said he gave him 'an expert's point of view' arising from a range of experience: 'obviously he'd seen a lot of cases and they could put it into the perspective of other cases he had seen'. One client, depressed and wishing to move house, commented on the enabling *encouragement* she'd got from the CPN, who refused simply to sympathize: 'it was come on, pull yourself together — pull yourself out of it. It was just what I needed'. What for others may have been insensitive was constructive for this client who, in retrospect, felt she had done insufficiently for herself.

Table 9.2 *Criticisms of Workers — Extended Intervention*

	Social Work	CPN
Relationship qualities	8	12
Expert skills	3	8
TOTAL	11	20

Criticisms of Workers

Table 9.2 shows a pattern by now familiar: CPNs performed worse than social workers. However, social workers were subject to a number of criticisms. Some involved relationship qualities. One client felt a *lack of genuine concern*:

> she was all right but quite a few times I was being treated by technique rather than as a genuine human being. I felt belittled by it.

Another client complained of *lack of openness* which had an impact on the pace of improvement: 'if she'd told me better what she thought I'd have been able to think about it more clearly and maybe be better informed about the future'. One client felt the worker could have shown *greater commitment*: in particular her timekeeping left something to be desired: 'I was there [at the Centre] and she wasn't and that was what mattered to me'. Other clients made complaints which were the reverse image of the commitment shown by a speedy response. One, with an appointment arranged by his GP complained 'I still had to wait half an hour' while another complained that 'it took about three weeks before they came' after the GP referred her and during that time her depression worsened. Another client, whose husband had left her within weeks of their marriage felt the waiting most strongly early in the intervention, when she was most vulnerable, although this became less important as she improved. This was similar to a man who had waited a week after referral, when he 'felt really bad' and needed a prompt response. One client questioned the *genuineness* of the worker who was concerned about her childrens' welfare, believing she made suggestions 'only to her [the worker's] advantage', and that her role impeded the genuine provision of advice:

> I feel as though she was governed by a responsibility of being a social worker. I think she felt frustrated that I wouldn't, or couldn't cooperate.

One client, experiencing marital difficulties, complained of *poor advice*: 'the only bit I didn't like was when she said if you can't cope with it just dump him'. The worker here had not appreciated her commitment to her partner. A failure to 'tune in' had led to advice which jarred with the woman. Two clients considered workers' abilities to *increase self understanding* were limited. One client felt the worker had listened but

> I was looking for more though. It's difficult to say what. Maybe an answer to why I drink. But it's not clear really. I wanted to stop.

Another woman, suffering periodic bouts of depression said,

> [social worker] is a social worker. I think I could probably have done with a psychiatrist — someone who could have dug deeper down to look properly at things. She helped me with immediate problems but I wanted to explore myself in more detail.

She had a touching faith in psychiatrists which may not have survived the first prescription of amitriptyline or course of ECT!

Criticisms of CPNs were more extensive and some were expressed in terms more emphatic than social workers. Some clients complained of a *lack of understanding*. A client suffering anxiety said

> I got the feeling that they were saying well 'yeah, yeah, I bet he's been like this all his life' and they didn't seem to give any credit for them being real problems.

Another depressed woman, both of whose parents had recently died, and finding it difficult to cope was told 'she was trying to opt out' when she wanted hospitalization 'to get over my grief ... and get away from the pressures that I couldn't cope with'. One woman, depressed by her run down flat in a deprived and vandalized area, said

> she could have been a little more understanding ... it's really people who've got semi-detached houses — they don't have these problems. When she told us about her housing problems she was a bit insensitive — the worst that seemed to happen to her was that the dog peed in the garden.

The CPN's response, for the client, indicated a supercilious lack of empathy. Another client, seeking to share her own experience of depression, suggested the CPN might find it difficult to understand having not experienced it herself. However the CPN's reply of 'how do you know?' left her very much 'up in the air' when she was seeking to be understood.

Other clients made criticisms betokening a perceived *lack of commitment*. One client with multiple problems additional to anxiety felt the CPN lost interest: 'she said she didn't feel I needed to go any more.... I felt quite discouraged by this.... I felt I'd like to have still gone to talk about other problems — like the one with my mum'. Another client complained that 'there were times when I felt I was shut up and bundled out of the door well before I should have been'. One client who was seeing both a psychiatrist and a CPN felt both were trying to palm him off on the other, and he was just going downhill: 'I felt as if I was being pushed from pillar to post and all help was just passing me by'. Other complaints included a lack of reliability: one CPN failed to see an anxious client despite having previously promised to contact him soon. After three weeks waiting the client went to the Centre himself. Another complaint was of a lack of consistency: after an initial visit a client was asked to return the next day:

> the nurse I saw spoke to me for ten minutes and said I'd already discussed this and that it wasn't worth going on. I was left feeling much worse that particular time.

Another client complained of the initial wait which was 'obviously discouraging'. One client with anxiety questioned the *genuineness* of the CPN because he could not 'often tell what he's thinking ... it's a bit like mind games and I'm not very good at them'. Another, not unintelligent, man felt a *lack of acceptance* and respect by the CPN: 'I did feel she belittled me. I felt a bit stupid by the way she talked'. This patronizing attitude questions the motives of the CPN for involvement, and the client wished he had seen a psychiatrist.

A number of criticisms related to expert skills. Three involved poor or non-existent advice. Two of these related to drugs. One, who was advised to discontinue taking tranquilizers because they would provide no solution, felt the nurse both stated the obvious and failed to understand the difficulties. Another client who had reduced his medication with the ultimate aim of dispensing with it was concerned about the attendant anxiety growth: 'he didn't even tell me whether my dreadful feelings were innate or whether they were drug withdrawal'. One man complained that the nurse seemed to think that just by talking the client would unburden himself 'but there were no constructive suggestions — no food for thought. Basically the things that were worrying me then are still worrying me now'.

Other complaints relate to analytic processes. One client felt a failure of assessment was directly related to a lack of appropriate intervention:

> he didn't seem to touch many areas. I was feeling very tense and anxious and no-one actually did anything to resolve it.

A woman who felt she was agoraphobic made a similar complaint. The agoraphobia was considered but 'there were a lot of other problems which weren't really touched'. One man was frustrated by the lack of appropriate analysis. He compared it with his own job (electrical diagnostician): 'if I have

Table 9.3   Impact of Workers' Involvement

	Social Work	CPNs
Worsened situation	—	1
No difference	4	7
Support at time only	2	2
Problem otherwise remained unresolved	2	4
Problem otherwise deteriorated	7	3
Improvement otherwise slowed	—	1
Possible suicide	3	1
No idea	1	—
TOTAL	19	19

a problem I look for the cause and cure it'. However, the CPN, he felt, made no attempt to get to the root of the problem. In the end he simply 'gave up coming because I didn't feel I was getting anything from it'. Complaints were not always about assessment. A woman with severe housing problems felt some tasks, particularly an attempt to get housing priority should have occurred: '[I] felt I could have been given some hope. She could have tried to contact housing to see what could be done'. This was a problem at root practical when talking only was on offer. Finally, one man felt the absence of a truly therapeutic response which would have helped self understanding of his severe emotional problems and the sense of futility he had.

> I would have liked the opportunity to go into the emotional stuff underlying the anxiety — things like my relations with my family, the feelings of futility at having wasted years in not being able to work.

The Impact of Workers

The other major issue confronted with clients was the difference intervention made to the client (table 9.3). As with other indicators the CPNs fared rather worse than social workers: in eight cases (42 per cent) CPN clients felt their intervention made no difference or worse, compared with only four (21 per cent) social work clients. These, like comments on skills give substance to the different levels of satisfaction between the two client groups. Among *social work* clients who felt intervention made no difference, two felt improvement occurred through their efforts, reflecting a lack of effective help by the worker. Two felt no improvement had occurred, one in their emotional state, the other in their housing problems. In both cases the client felt there was little the worker *could* have done to help. Two clients felt supported because there was someone other than their family to turn to. The most dramatic effects of intervention were on those who considered possible suicide. One said

> I think I would have took another overdose. I suppose . . . I felt at the time that nobody cared.

Another also said she could have overdosed, while a third said the worker 'stopped me killing myself'.

Those who considered they would have deteriorated were at times also dramatic. Some considered their mental health state would have worsened. One said

> I think I would have got more depressed — got worse. It's not the kind of thing you like to think about really.

Others said they would have been 'worse and much iller' or 'the anxieties would have been worse'. Others were more general:

> I think I would have cracked and that. I'm not saying I would have took tablets and become suicidal, but I think I wouldn't have been able to cope.

One client said 'I would have been a bit more isolated . . . more into myself', another said things 'were going to get worse. Drinking in particular and work' and a woman with marital problems said 'I don't think I would have been here now. I would have left him and not come back. We would have just separated. Things were so bad I just couldn't see any way out'. Even those who suggested the problem would have remained indicated how significant intervention could be. One woman, sexually abused by her father as a teenager, said

> a lot. For one, I wouldn't have sorted myself. Things would have dragged on. I needed to talk. I needed to bring things out into the open which I couldn't do before.

Another considered she would have remained depressed by her marital difficulties.

Among *CPN* clients, the one whose situation was worsened achieved this through a reduction of hope: 'in the long run I felt a bit let down — of not being taken seriously and not given much help.' If after seeking professional help the CPNs were no use, who would be? There were various reasons why intervention made no difference. In two cases clients were disparaging about CPN skills. One client considered intervention was primarily limited to listening, which 'didn't seem to improve things in the long run', while another said in relation to skills: 'I don't think it made any difference at all — there was little constructive at all'. Another client said he was already receiving help from social services (although this was only a home help). CPNs would not normally see their skills interchangeable with those of home helps. One man attributed their limited effect to the lateness of the referral and that consequently much improvement had already occurred before intervention. Two clients felt that the nature of their problems were such that they would have to take their course — intervention would make little difference — while one felt that they had the inner strength to cope with their problems, although visits were 'something to look forward to'. These variations show that the 'no difference' response meant different things to clients, although while some were disparaging, none indicated a noticeably positive perception of the CPN's impact.

Those who cited support at the time as the main impact also demonstrated variations. Hence the tone of one client: 'it did have a short term immediate effect . . . it did ease the situation at the time' was less enthusiastic than that of another client who subsequently discovered she was seriously ill:

I don't know how I'd have got through those months. I was feeling really ill and they could not find anything wrong at the time. He also took my mind off immediate problems.

Other clients felt their problems would have remained unresolved. One agoraphobic woman said she would probably have reached the stage where 'I could not go outside the door', while a depressed woman, not eating or sleeping 'would still have been in that position'. Two women had marital problems: one felt she 'would have gone round and round in circles without sorting it out' while the other felt 'it would have taken a lot to get myself out of it'. Others felt their situation would have deteriorated, as with one client who felt they 'would have had a nervous breakdown', another with marital problems who said 'I think I'd probably be on my own now' and a further client who could only see themselves 'going downhill'. One client felt their improvement would have been slower, 'she put a spurt on it', while another who lost his wife and child said 'I might have committed suicide. I don't know. He helped me face the situation'.

Comments

The analysis of extended intervention shows in a number of respects differences from brief intervention. First, the average number of skills per client evident from clients' accounts is greater, for both CPNs and social workers than with brief intervention. This is evident with both relationship qualities and expert skills. Furthermore, a wider range of expert skills, particularly amongst social work clients is evident with extended intervention. This is perhaps not surprising, though it may reflect a number of possibilities. The nature of the work, differing from brief intervention, may require a greater range of skills. Alternatively the greater amount of time available may allow the workers actually to display a greater range of skills. It may simply reflect, furthermore, a greater opportunity for clients simply to *experience* these skills, that is, with a longer period of time, they become more aware of their use. Finally, it may reflect a combination of two or more of these alternatives. The average number of criticisms of skills per client was rather lower with extended than brief intervention. For social workers these averaged 0.69 per client for brief intervention compared with 0.57 for extended intervention. For CPNs they averaged 1.46 with brief intervention and 1.05 with extended intervention. This, then, serves to emphasize the impression left by clients' comments on skills: that they experienced a greater level of overall skills than clients receiving brief intervention.

However in one important respect, the clients' experience of extended intervention is similar to that of brief intervention: both CPN and social work clients identified considerably more relationship qualities than expert skills. This indicates, as with brief intervention, that the human qualities of caring, empathy, listening and so on were highly prized by the clients. This is stated with the caveat, noted earlier, that clients may find greater difficulty identifying, or giving expression to, the expert skills. However, although this overall position holds for both brief and extended intervention, detailed analysis shows interesting differences. The *ratio* of relationship qualities to expert skills was 3:1 for social workers undertaking brief intervention, but only 1.9:1 for extended intervention. Expert skills, therefore, had a relatively higher profile in these clients' experience of extended intervention. However, the reverse was the case with CPNs. The ratio of relationship qualities to expert skills was, for brief intervention, 2.4:1 but for extended intervention 3.0:1. This is particularly interesting in view of the wider range of expert skills identified by social work, compared with CPN, clients receiving extended intervention.

Other differences are evident between CPNs and social workers, and these are again in line with much of the other evidence. Social work clients identified a greater number of skills than CPN clients and this involved both relationship qualities and expert skills. Social work clients also made fewer criticisms of skills than CPN clients, and this also was the case with both relationship qualities and expert skills. Taken together with the evidence presented elsewhere in the book, it appears overall to make a considerable difference for clients as to which of these two occupations they are allocated.[1] Clients' responses, with extended intervention, to the question about the impact of the workers' involvement show social workers less frequently made no difference or worsened the situation, and, most dramatically, more frequently prevented possible suicide. These responses, finally, indicate something of major importance for practice: that intervention can, at times, from the client's perspective, not simply help, but have an enormous impact. It is most obvious with the aversion of possible suicides, but comments by other clients give ample evidence of their great impact. Furthermore, to the extent that these comments were more consistently made about social workers, they can take considerable satisfaction from this. David Howe (1980) has suggested, with some justification, that social workers should show more humility, particularly in their claims arising from their professional knowledge base. These results suggest, nonetheless, that they might show greater confidence, and less self criticism, about the potential impact of their help.

Note

1 Of course, as previously noted clients make judgments in the context of their experiences elsewhere. Indeed some writers emphasize (see for example, Fisher, 1983) the social context against which background assumptions develop. These will, no doubt have influenced these clients' responses. However, it appears extremely unlikely that these results arose primarily because of different background assumptions. For this to be the case:

1 these assumptions would have had to make clients consistently and systematically better disposed towards social workers;
2 their impact would have had to have been sufficient to override the actual behaviour of the professionals;
3 this would have had to persist over both brief *and* extended work; and
4 it would have had to be maintained over quantitative as well as qualitative measures.

Chapter 10

Conclusions

Role and Skills

It is now possible to draw together some key elements of social workers' and CPNs' practice. Of course these observations relate to a CMHC setting. Although each will have distinctive characteristics, this was a particularly good example since it was both well established and possessed many elements characterizing CMHCs as a whole. Additionally, its emphasis on neurotic, emotional and relationship problems reflects the known extent of minor mental illness in general population studies. It exemplifies, therefore, two elements which may be expected to characterize significant elements of community care: an extensive clientele with minor mental illness and emotional problems, and a CMHC base.

It is first evident that for social workers brief intervention seemed to limit their range of work compared with extended intervention. Brief work most noticeably involved greater emphasis on mental health cases, work at the non-health community-agency level was more restricted, although greater than CPN or joint intervention, a greater proportion of problems were not tackled, and they noticeably undertook little psychodynamic work. CPNs, on the other hand displayed fewer differences between brief and extended work. CPNs displayed a greater emphasis than social workers, with both brief and extended intervention, on mental health cases. Like social workers, CPN extended cases were more complex than brief cases with more severe social problems and problems per case. With extended intervention anxiety had by far the highest profile of primary problems. Both brief and extended intervention were characterized by work with the client alone, although they contacted non-health community-agencies even *less* with extended than brief intervention. For social workers, a greater emphasis with extended intervention on social problem cases was accompanied by a philosophy of intervention whereby social workers undertook more interviews and displayed a greater intensity of work than CPNs, together with a strong emphasis on psychodynamic work and emotional support. Although they showed a greater propensity than CPNs to work with practical problems, this may have been less than it could have been, suggesting *at times*, a counselling rather than casework role.

It appears, to a considerable degree, that with brief intervention the two occupations are interchangeable, indicating for this work the advent of the 'mental health worker'. Little benefit, though, appeared to arise from joint work. However, this work was very brief, and very often was only assessment followed by referral to other agencies. With extended work differences are clear. CPNs were strongly oriented to individualist work; they concentrated, though not exclusively, on mental health cases, and these were primarily neurotic, particularly anxiety; their cases were significantly less complex than social workers; they undertook a more limited range of roles, and little psychodynamic work; when contacting outside agencies and professionals these were mainly health (primarily doctors). Social workers, on the other hand, worked mainly with social problem cases: their work stressed the area of neurotic/emotional/relationship problems; their cases were significantly more complex than CPNs', and problems were more severe; they worked in a far wider context than CPNs; their roles were wider, and they showed a philosophy of intervention in which psychodynamic work and emotional support in combination played a major part; and they contacted a wider range of outside agencies and professionals. These are clearly quite separate professional groups with a division of labour and style of work displaying marked differences.

Skills analysis also indicates major differences. With brief intervention joint work does not involve an accretion of skills. Indeed, like CPNs, they generally perform less impressively than social workers. Apart from problem identification, therefore, there is little support for the superiority of joint over individual (social) work. Overall clients were most satisfied with social work. Except with brief mental health problems social work clients showed a greater awareness of their worker's definition of social and mental health problems. Social work clients were more aware of their problem definition, and more accurately identified activities undertaken than CPN clients. CPN clients saw them as more passive than social workers in defining, planning and carrying out intervention, and more frequently would have preferred alternative activities. Compared with their clients CPNs showed a more exaggerated perception of positive change than social workers. Social work clients, with both brief and extended intervention identified far more skills, both relationship and expert, than CPN clients. Criticisms of CPNs, skills were greater overall than social work skills, while social work clients felt least frequently that intervention made no difference, while social workers generally seemed to have a greater impact. With extended work in particular, social workers displayed a wider range of expert skills, noticeably analytic processes, information, release of feelings and increasing self understanding. The latter two are interesting, as psychodynamic skills, while clients also more frequently found social workers were empathic, listened and gave support.

How widely may these observations, particularly those related to CPN role and skills, be applied? Although focusing on particular teams, there are reasons to believe this study has wide implications. The first is the theory practice relationship, discussed in more detail later. Although the results are complex, there are many respects in which the extent and limits of theory are produced in practice. If theory does have an impact on practice, and this is discussed later, then the limits of theory are liable to be reproduced by social workers and CPNs working elsewhere. Second, however, we can relate this to evidence gained elsewhere. Sladden (1979) who studied hospital based CPNs in Edinburgh found that in non-clinical domains nurses found difficulty in defining situations needs and problems in terms of general concepts which could be used as a basis for rational selection of methods of care and evaluation of results. Psychosocial nursing practice seemed to be based on a rather haphazard application of intuitive insights and individual experience. Second, where relationship difficulties existed — and they were extensive — the nurses appeared able to identify and describe these situations, but they were often at a loss as to how to deal with them. Relationship problems within families were found most problematic, leaving nurses with feelings of frustration and inadequacy. Indeed Sladden commented both that psychiatrists tended to view CPNs as second rate psychotherapists, and that the possibility of involving social workers did not appear to be considered by CPNs. Finally, clinical assessment and observation took precedence over psychosocial aspects of work. With interpersonal work nurses often provided support, but primarily in the form of a sort of social visiting whose principle object was to provide social contact for people. When faced with a change in the patient they tended to resort to a medical frame of reference rather than seek precipitants in family relationships or social environment.

The other major study is Wooff's (1987). Having undertaken theory analysis, we are in a better position to view her findings. Her CPNs were based in a primary care setting. Their practice appeared more haphazard than social workers': they called upon clients without prior arrangement, they did not feel it necessary to structure their time with clients, and they did not receive regular support and supervision. Second, CPNs were less committed to the concept of teamwork than social workers, preferring single handed direct contact with clients. She observed (though did not measure in her study) a considerable amount of contact by social workers, unlike CPNs, with outside organizations. Finally while CPNs provided technical clinical skills, they displayed a relative lack of counselling and therapeutic skills. More often they discussed methods of coping with symptoms and behaviour, frequently inviting clients to attend relaxation groups and advised the use of relaxation tapes. Social work discussions were more wide ranging involving family and welfare issues.

These studies were undertaken in geographically separate parts of the country, and, interestingly, in separate settings: Sladden's CPNs were hospital based, and Wooff's were primary care based. Yet our framework allows us to identify common factors. First, CPNs appear less able (if at all) to operate at the community agency level, and indeed display noticeable individualist approaches; second, their ability to use therapeutic approaches appears limited; third, they appear more uncomfortable managing relationship problems (hence working with more than one client); and fourth, they have less ability to adopt a wide ranging psychosocial approach to problems. Our research, based on a CMHC, concentrated most on neurotic, emotional and relationship problems and hence focused most strongly on the psychosocial (rather than bio) domain, one claimed by both occupations. Our detailed analysis of theory shows that these factors common to these studies reflect the range and comprehensiveness of these occupations' theory base.

Theory and Practice

This study has been characterized by a dual focus on theory and practice. These may of course be studied separately and on this basis conclude CPNs appear less developed than social work in both areas. A connection was created through the methodology (see Appendix 1 to this volume) in which the instruments used to examine practice were, to a great degree, derived from theory. What was not examined was the *process* by which theory was transmitted into practice. Taken at face value evidence of some connections appear strong — there is considerable apparent symmetry between theory and practice — and some comments may usefully be made. We may tentatively outline some of the main issues which might explain some connections. This will focus on the creation of perspectives through education and training on one hand, and the limits to these provided by agency setting on the other.

Atkinson (1983) emphasizes the importance of influence provided by the transmission of knowledge on the behaviour of professions, and the reproduction of that behaviour in 'new' professionals. He advocates examining 'the relationship between education, practice and the organization of occupational groups'. The knowledge and education of the profession will help develop characteristic traits in members of that profession. He emphasizes that knowledge is not simple, objective and uncontroversial but, through curriculum and values is classified and combined in certain ways — it is a cultural imposition. To the extent that CPNs and social workers differ in the content of their education they will possess different cultures.

Bernstein (1971, 1975) suggests that educational knowledge is a major regulator of the structure of experience. Education is not merely that which is formally taught, but may be acquired through reading professionally relevant literature, which may occur in practice and long after formal courses of training. He uses Durkheim's concept of 'boundary maintenance' in order to examine the separation and differentiation of categories or areas of knowledge. Although working with ideal types, he suggests knowledge may be segmented into categories, each of which is highly separate from others, or the boundaries may be blurred, and separation between different 'bits' of knowledge would be correspondingly reduced, to a point ultimately where they could be integrated. He uses the terms collection code and integrated code to identify these two tendencies, which represent extreme ends of a spectrum.

This is significant because it suggests that the knowledge base of a profession will exercise a major influence on the way its members experience and define the world — what they perceive their world to be, what is noticed and what is not, what is ascribed with importance, and what is not dignified with a passing thought. Where boundary maintenance is strong this can have a significant influence. Social work, emphasizing a social science knowledge base has long experienced difficulty relating to the medical profession, with its emphasis on the natural sciences, physiology, anatomy and so on. Indeed, the 'behavioural sciences' newly introduced into the medical curriculum sits uneasily with its natural science knowledge base (Walton, 1984).

The knowledge base or perspective, then, may be expected to influence significantly the forms of behaviour characteristic of occupations. However, the *raison d'etre* for professional knowledge is its practice use: it is applied rather than pure in nature. This raises a number of relevant issues. First, not all situations confronting practitioners are known. Jamous and Pelioille (1970) refer to this in terms of technicality — methods which may be transmitted and mastered in the form of rules — and indetermination — those which cannot, and emphasize the individual qualities (virtualities) of the practitioner. The position any problem occupies on the technicality-indetermination spectrum will determine the importance of experience or personal qualities as compared with learned knowledge. A second element relates to the attitude of the professionals involved. Medicine has, according to Freidson (1970) a strong body of knowledge which is not always utilized. Medicine values the qualities of individuals who practice, resulting, he suggests, in a tendency to emphasize the indeterminacy and uncertainty of the phenomena with which practitioners deal, at the expense of regularity and lawful scientific behaviour in their practice. 'Real Medicine' is to be learned at the patient's bedside, learning through actual experience, thus emphasizing the superiority of experience over theory (the 'clinical gaze'). Atkinson (1977) calls this 'training for dogmatism', where professionals assert the correctness of (their) personal experience, even in the face of extensive and contradictory empirical evidence. The third element is a difficulty of 'fit' between the theory and its application to practice. In this case relevant knowledge is available, but its application by the professional to particular individual circumstances requires some imagination and flexibility on their part (Merton *et al.*, 1957).

Two further issues may be considered from occupational sociology. Pavalko (1971) identifies two significant aspects of training. The first is theory: the extent to which there is a systematic body of theory and esoteric abstract knowledge on which work is based. This body of knowledge is the basis for the professional's claim to expertise. Second, the training period is significant. This involves four factors: the amount of training which is involved, the extent to which it is specialized, the degree to which it is symbolic and ideational, and the content of what is learned during the training period (the distinctive set of values, norms and work role conceptions as well as specific knowledge and skills). The greater the extent of these four factors, the stronger will be the occupation's claim to uniqueness (and professional status). Simpson (1967) identified three major stages through which the individual shifts their attention from the broad societally derived goals which led them to choose the profession to the point where he internalizes the skills and values of the group and adopts the behaviour it prescribes. However, socialization (and learning) does not end with training. Control may be exercised by formal means, such as codes of ethics, or by more informal means, which includes colleague evaluation. In professions emphasizing a service ethic, approval of work by colleagues can become a critical measure of success. Where individuals are strongly identified with their occupational group, the seeking of colleague approval gives colleagues a high degree of control over an individual's behaviour (Fichter, 1961). Second, loyalty may be focused on the organization, where the reference group against which an individual judges his performance lies *within* the organization, or cosmopolitan, primarily involving orientation to an outside reference group representing a professional specialty (Gouldner, 1957).

This is a schematic outline of some major factors likely to exert an influence on the theory — practice relationship. These may be presented thus:

Knowledge	Technical	Indeterminate
Boundary Maintenance	Collection	Integrated
Attitudes	Collective	Person Centred
	(Common Skills)	(Virtualities)
Training	Extensive	Limited
Post Training	Profession	Organization (colleague)
	orientation	orientation.

Each of these may be presented as extreme ends of a spectrum. Those on the left would *tend* to induce professional uniqueness and differentiation between occupations. The doctor working with the social worker may emphasize this in relation to biophysical knowledge. That tending to the right where knowledge is more indeterminate, that which exists is generally integrated, personal qualities are emphasized will tend to create overlaps between occupations (overlaps may also be created where knowledge and skills are similar).

There is some evidence of boundary maintenance in the research, most obvious in relation to the context for intervention. Discussion of theory noted that claims by nurses to a domain including the psychosocial (as well as bio) was not matched by detailed development of approaches informing work in corresponding contexts. This was most evident with work on the social environment, an arena where social work has displayed considerable theoretical development, contrasting strongly with the individualist orientation of nursing. The boundary for CPNs is less between two separate areas of knowledge than between an area of knowledge (focusing on the individual) and none at all (focusing on the social environment). This led to claims in the domain of nursing (biopsychosocial) which were difficult to sustain in practice. Hence social workers operated considerably more extensively at the community agency level than CPNs. This suggests that boundaries set by theory acted as a constraint on practice: the social work community-agency orientation and its lack amongst CPNs reflected their respective occupational theory.

Analysis of theory, however, showed it was less characterized by strict boundaries between knowledge adopted by CPNs and social workers. Rather they display either different foci or different degrees of sophistication. An example of the former is a CPN knowledge organized around models of mental illness, and social work's social science-knowledge base. Each does not exclude the other but they place differing emphasis on the definition of their work. Differing sophistication over the same area is evident in the analysis of interpersonal skills, where nursing is less integrated in its approach. In practice we see a greater emphasis by CPNs on mental health cases and social workers on social problem cases. Equally CPNs were not devoid of interpersonal skills. They were simply displayed more sporadically, noticeably less in expert skills, and with greater client reservations. If a theory-practice relationship exists, therefore, it appears as a predisposing influence, with workers tending to adopt behaviour reflecting theory rather than slavishly following it. Differences are nonetheless significant.

The extent to which the knowledge base is technical or indeterminate and to which personal flair at the application of particular approaches is significant appear closely related. We are not discussing extremes. Rather as both professions emphasize there is a personal judgment dimension to practice: we are, therefore, discussing the *degree* of influence theory has on practice. If practice were entirely based on practitioners' personal qualities explanations for differences between occupations would not require recourse to their theory base. The results, however, seem to indicate something more than this. Practitioners may not be able to claim that if they apply approach A to problem B outcome C will occur but the 'contours' of practice, the emphasis placed by practitioners on different approaches and definitions of their work, display a remarkable, if imperfect, reflection of theory. We might anyway not expect the reflection to be precise. This first relates to the limits of theory in its ability to control situations of concern to practice, and hence the significance of personal qualities. It second relates to an oversocialized conception of humans. Humans are conscious beings who assess, interpret and define their circumstances. It is a mistake to believe that socialization *determines* the way we act: humans have the ability to act back and exercise some choice (particularly as adults) about what they 'take on board'.

The relative influence of training and post training experience is an issue. CPNs in the psychosocial realm possess a relatively limited and fragmentary theory base compared with social workers. Social work theory may not be able to predict that approach A applied to problem B will yield outcome C. It does, though, provide ways of working in an uncertain professional world by providing ways of understanding individuals, families and groups in their social context, and flexibility, the preparedness to use different constructs and approaches as situations require is the hallmark of the imaginative social worker. The more restricted fragmentary CPN psychosocial theory base is again shown in the example of intervention context: their individualist orientation not giving them the range of possible alternatives available to social workers whose theories provide them with a more unified conception of moving between contexts. The suggestion, then, is that theory (hence training) has an impact on practice. What of post training experience? It is possible following training to develop a more practice orientated use of theory by working through different perspectives and approaches through exposure to practice situations. At least two factors additional to initial training may be significant — the growth of experience through exposure to practice situations and the impact of colleague consultation and guidance (e.g. through discussion or supervision). This raises questions of who is regarded as colleagues and of 'seepage' of theories or approaches between occupations. All the workers were experienced and had the opportunity to consolidate their respective professional learning prior to CMHC involvement. However, the agency claimed that working from the same base facilitated the crossover of ideas and practice. This could take two forms: discussion of cases formally (e.g. in allocation) or informally (on an ad hoc basis), or through joint work. The opportunity existed, therefore, for seepage. Some of this may have occurred, differences might have been even more marked. But the consistency with which differences persisted over a variety of measures indicates a certain robustness about these occupational differences: their work suggests ideas and practices did not cross easily between occupations. Overall, given the auspicious circumstances for role blurring and seepage, this research casts grave doubt on the possibility of the community mental health worker. Two bases for this: an overlap of theory and close working relations did not produce similar professionals.

This admittedly schematic outline has introduced concepts aiding understanding of theory-practice relationships. Howe (1986) has suggested, however, that examining social work with reference only to 'professional' social work concepts frustrates creating wider links between practice and the organization of social workers. He suggested fieldworkers and welfare managers represent two groups employing different strategies to establish control over work done. Control was represented as the extent to which workers' skills have a predictable effect on the ways clients are perceived and understood, and responses offered in the light of these perceptions. He found occupational skills generally failed to bring people and their situations under sufficient control. In these circumstances the more restricted strategies of managers and administrators were employed, and in their narrower definitions control could be more easily exercised. He suggested a close relationship between the weakness of social workers' expertise and the control exercised by managers, through authority based directives or by managerial design and structure. Where, for example, teenagers committed offences, discretion allowed social workers was withdrawn, and procedural guidelines or management directives held sway.

This study has not examined the intrusion of managerial power on professional practice. However, certain comments may be made. First our study compares two occupations: it may be that taking this (occupationally) wider view throws into sharper relief the more distinctively professional, as opposed to managerial, dimension of practice. Second, unlike Howe's social workers, based in area teams, these were specialists based in a health setting. It may be that, particularly in view of their closeness to medicine with its independent professional ethos, the tradition of psychiatric social work has emphasized greater practitioner's autonomy. Reference to the 'higher' authority of the consultant may occur in specific circumstances, e.g. a psychosis, which experienced workers might be expected to recognize easily. It should be noted, of course, that the service was not medically controlled. Third, client responses suggest that, for them, a high degree of control was established either by stabilizing their situation, preventing deterioration, or improvement. In a sense, the issue is who defines (clients, manager, politicians) when control is achieved? Certainly many clients felt some control was achieved. Fourth, this work may be different from, say, juvenile offenders or child abuse. It might be regarded as less sensitive and crucial and hence less subject to managerial control. Finally, the ultimate sanction in mental health lay with practitioners themselves: as approved social workers they could compulsorily admit some people. Hence, when control was failing, the focus was likely to remain on the practitioner rather than manager.

Knowledge and Training

In recent years there has been some debate on the status of the social work knowledge base (Davies, 1981, 1982, 1986; Hardiker, 1981; Sibeon, 1982). It is unnecessary to repeat this debate, to which I have contributed (Sheppard, 1984; 1990), in detail. In brief it involves issues of *whether* social science is relevant to social work practice, and if so *how* it may be applied. Those emphasizing its limitations have done so basically on three grounds: that the nature of the social sciences are such that they are riven with contradictions and inconsistencies which make them an unsafe foundation for practice (Howe, 1980); that when apparently relevant elements of knowledge (such as attachment and bonding) are available, far more pervasive influences on what social workers do are exercised by the constraints of practice, such as limited resources; and finally, that sociology (or parts thereof) has exercised a nefarious influence on those training for social work, potentially undermining their commitment to practice (Davies, 1986). Others have disputed this, suggesting that social sciences are multiparadigmatic, and some elements dovetail easily with social work; that social work theory is steeped in social science perspectives, which cannot be surgically removed; that social workers *do* use conceptual frameworks which have an impact on practice (Hardiker, 1981; Sibeon, 1982).

Although the debate has generally been of a high standard, it is not always clear in which sense social science may be conceived. On the one hand there are what may be broadly termed 'theories of understanding': theoretical and empirical information which helps understanding of the nature, cause, process and outcome of social phenomena (e.g. depression, juvenile offending). On the other hand there are what may be broadly termed 'theories of helping': those which provide social work with alternative ways of managing the problems with which they are concerned (e.g. task centred, problem solving, systems). Thus Davies concerns himself largely with the former while Sheldon (1978) concerns himself primarily with the latter. However, separation is far from complete: both are concerned with social phenomena and the social world. Theories of understanding (e.g. on social networks and support) may in part underpin theories of helping (e.g. ecological approaches), while the language used in theories of helping is consistently that of the social world. Furthermore evaluations of the effectiveness of theories of helping (e.g. Gibbons *et al.*, 1978, 1979) provide a contribution to the understanding of social phenomena (what happens when social workers behave in particular ways) which may later contribute to its explanation.

Although, therefore, we may separate these theory types by their focus (on understanding or helping) complete differentiation is not possible. The social work theory base, as discussed in Chapters 2 and 6 involves the use of perspectives based on a broad concentration on the social world. A number of relevant points may be made about these. First as we have already noted, judgment of the social work theory base is better undertaken by comparison with relevant alternatives rather than erecting some idealized standard for comparison. On this basis its theory stands up well to that of CPNs. Second, there is good reason to believe it exercises a strong influence on actual practice, which we have discussed. Third, on the basis of clients' views, evidence suggests social workers performed rather better than CPNs (who did not have recourse to the social work theory base). Elsewhere, I have begun to develop principles which may help theories of understanding to become more relevant to *assessment* in practice situations (Sheppard 1984, 1990). This study has suggested that existing approaches, to a considerable degree involving intervention rather than just assessment, have an impact on practice.

The central issues for CPNs are somewhat different, and perhaps more fundamental. CPNs have not engaged in a detailed debate of the sort undertaken by social workers on the nature and relevance of their knowledge base. Indeed it may be insufficiently coherent to allow such a debate to develop. Their major concerns relate to the training of psychiatric nurses for the community role, particularly the community qualification (ENB 810, 811, 812), which lasts nine months. Although no CPNs in this study had this qualification, it should be noted at the outset that only a small minority (between 20 and 30 per cent) of CPNs nationally hold this qualification.[1] The CPNs in this study, therefore, are representative in this respect of the vast majority in Britain. This will probably remain the case for the forseeable future. First, the proportion of CPNs with this qualification has remained fairly steady in the 1980s. Second, the qualification is not itself mandatory (and it is difficult to see how it could be when only a quarter *are* so qualified). Third, there is a shortage of financial support by health authorities limiting the number seconded.

These data, then are about nurses with representative qualifications rather than wishful thinking about community qualified CPNs. Furthermore, claims by CPNs to roles similar to social workers would require the development of appropriate skills and approaches on these courses. How realistic is this? Any changes induced by this training would certainly on our evidence have to be dramatic. Evidence on this is sparse, but largely discouraging. One study has suggested community training (at Sheffield Polytechnic) did have an effect (Brooker, 1990). Based on the views of nurses completing training and their managers, Brooker felt both groups considered improvements had occurred in clinical practice, knowledge base and initiating changes, although in contradiction nearly half the nurses felt the course had not met their major expectation, particularly in clinical skills. Notwithstanding this, these are simply general views: we have already shown how clients may have a less optimistic view of CPN practice than CPNs themselves. Second, it is not based on case by case analysis of actual practice: we cannot therefore evaluate its effect on practice. Wooff *et al.* (1988a) who did do this, admittedly only with a small group of CPNs, found no discernable differences between the work of 'trained' and 'untrained' CPNs.

Other studies, primarily of CPNs' views, are equally pessimistic. Skidmore and Friend (1984), comparing (of 120 cohorts) the 40 per cent who had taken the ENB course with those who had not, concluded (with little comment) that there were no significant differences between these groups in nursing care effectiveness. Work methods were developed more by trial and error than logical progression. Second, there has been concern over the relatively static and academic manner in which courses have been taught. There has been widespread consensus that such courses should be skills based and reflect the CPNs' work context (Reed, 1988). The problem has been seen as the combination of theory and practice: theory should be reflected in practice rather than standing alone. This may, though, be a misrepresentation of the problem. The theory itself may be inadequate. Our evidence suggests the theory-practice gap arises not because of too academic an approach, but because of the *limitations* of theory available to CPNs. For this gap to be bridged access is required to appropriate theory: the need for counselling skills is at times mentioned, although those of social casework and community social work appear most appropriate — precisely those skills characteristic of social work. Third, emphasis should be on effective practice, and assessment criteria should reflect this (Skidmore, 1985): like other practice based disciplines emphasis should be on supervised practice as a learning medium. But who is to do this? Only a quarter of CPNs are community qualified (and many are apparently dubious about its use). ENB regulations (811, 812) do not require supervisors to be community qualified, only that they are 'appropriately qualified and experienced mental health nurses'. Thus, while they are confronted on one hand with a theory-practice divide, increased emphasis on practice supervision is liable to involve 'the blind leading the blind'. Indeed, an emphasis on practice learning must make us dubious of a qualification which can be obtained through distance learning (Rushforth, 1990).

CPNs may be described as the 'artful dodgers' of the mental health world. They have expanded only by stealing roles previously belonging to other occupations without quite knowing what to do when they have them. If, perhaps simplistically, we equate 'bio' primarily with medical skills, 'psycho' with psychologists and 'psychosocial' with social workers it is difficult to see where room exists for CPNs. They may learn behavioural methods, but they then operate essentially as behavioural psychologists. They may expand to fill gaps left by PSWs, but they have failed to develop the knowledge and skills appropriate to this task. As a result the need for counselling skills is emphasized (Skidmore, 1985; ENB, 1989) and even casework skills are mentioned (CPNA, 1985a). These are tacit admissions that nursing does not possess a theory base adequate to the task. They present as a largely theory-less (or limited) occupation desperately seeking an appropriate theory base. Health Service managers may reasonably ask: why bother to invest finances in such a dubious enterprise as post qualification training? After all social workers on the evidence of this study *already possess* the skills sought by CPNs. Resources might more effectively be sent (though Social Services) in that direction. However, the momentum created by occupational ambition and expansion makes it unlikely that CPNs will retreat to the more limited clinical support role of earlier days.

Final Comment: Case Management

Following the publication in 1989 of the White Paper on Community Care, a great emphasis has been placed on case management. This is new to this country but is fairly well established in the United States. It appears primarily directed at chronically mentally disabled patients, who constitute a small proportion of this study, but the *methods* of case management have some relevance. In state programmes, case managers are viewed not necessarily as service providers themselves, but as case coordinators and personal service brokers who expedite clients through various services to which they are entitled (Johnson and Rubin, 1983). Their work involves assessment of individuals, planning, linking clients to formal and informal care systems and service provision, monitoring the clients' progress and advocacy on behalf of the client. The key to this is the ability easily to operate with community agencies and support systems. Johnson and Rubin (1983), American authors, suggest that current conceptual frameworks for social work practice, with their underlying focus on person in environment interface, suggest a compelling case for social work leadership. Although we have noted occasions where, in this study, social workers may manifest insufficient concern for practical issues, they appear incomparably better equipped than CPNs for case management. Indeed Johnson and Rubin (1983) suggest the broker of services role is appropriately allied to the primary therapist role with the clients and the person who works with the family. This range of work fits better, both in theory and practice, with social work. Social work, therefore, appear best suited for developments in community care leading up to and into the next century.

Note

1   At the time of writing, data from the latest CPNA survey were not available. Ted White of Manchester University, who has been collating these data, suggested that early results indicate that the proportion of CPNs holding the ENB 810 and 811 community qualification my have risen since 1985 by about 5 to 8 per cent. It remains highly probable that for the foreseeable future the overwhelming majority of CPNs will not hold this, or the ENB 812, qualification.

Methodology

This study had two aspects: a survey of referrals to the WIS undertaken with the workers and interviews with a sample of clients. The chronology of research was as follows:

1 December 1987 to 31 March 1988: study of all referrals made to the WIS, providing the basis for survey data and brief intervention data.

1 December 1987 to 31 November 1988: study of all clients allocated for extended intervention.

11 April 1988 to 17 February 1989: interviews with clients.

31 May 1989: research ceases (six months after allocation of final case).

The central theme of the approach to research made in this study was that it should be undertaken in terms meaningful to professionals involved. Another was that it involved triangulation: the use of different methods based on the belief that the combination of methods is superior to the use of a single method. Denzin (1978, p. 303) identifies four types of triangulation; within methods (involving replication), investigator triangulation (involving two or more investigators) between methods, and data triangulation. The latter two were used in this study. Data triangulation involves using more than one source of information (e.g. clients and workers), allowing for multiple perspectives, and method triangulation is based on the view that different methods have different strengths and weaknesses. This, it is believed, makes it more likely (though not certain) that an accurate representation of the phenomena under consideration is achieved (Smith, 1975; Hammersley and Atkinson, 1983).

The method triangulation involved a combination of survey and qualitative interview techniques. One facet of the distinction frequently drawn between quantitative and qualitative research is that the former tends to be oriented to the specific concerns of the investigator and the latter to the subjects' perspectives (Brymon, 1988). However, Marsh (1982) draws attention to the capacity of surveys to provide insights into questions of meaning, e.g. the widespread tendency among social researchers to solicit their respondents' reasons for their actions, views, etc., giving the example of Brown and Harris's (1978) effort to understand the meaning of life events to respondents in explaining depression. This may be placed in reverse: one problem with qualitative research is its tendency to rely on illustrative or anecdotal methods, through the use of quotes or descriptive work. Silverman (1985, p. 140) who is strongly committed to qualitative research commented that 'the critical reader is forced to ponder whether the researcher has selected only those fragments of data which support their argument', intentionally or otherwise. He suggests the use of simple counting techniques which allow the qualitative researcher to survey their data and to provide the reader with an overall impression of their data.

Data triangulation involved responses from both worker and client, the latter involving direct interviews by the researcher. Conspicuously missing from this triangulation was direct observation of worker client interviews. Its value is the ability to collect rich detailed data based on observations in natural settings (Burgess, 1984). However, it had crucial disadvantages. Most important were ethical: it presented the possibility that the provision of help would become secondary to the requirements of research. Also it is difficult to see how genuine permission could be provided by clients who may have agreed to the researcher's presence simply because they were so desperate to get help where they assumed agreement was necessary to get help. Second, the researcher's presence may have disrupted interviews, providing an alternative focus, present but not involved in the actual helping process. Third, there was the entirely practical reason that permission would not have been granted by the agency on this basis, for the two reasons already given.

Gaining Access

Access to professionals, agencies or data generally involve gatekeepers, key personnel who may grant or withhold access. (Hammersley and Atkinson, 1983). Access to this agency was a protracted process. Initial contact was with the district manager for hospital social work in June 1986, followed by contact with the senior social worker (mental health) and senior CPN (general psychiatry) responsible for the centre's work. Although the senior social worker was immediately interested, the senior CPN understandably voiced concerns, expressed primarily in terms of its drain on time and resources of the centre's personnel. Nonetheless both agreed to preliminary developments of questionnaires. However, developments were halted because of imminent changes in social service departmental structure and personnel which, it was felt, would disrupt research. The two seniors were again approached in May 1987. Although maintaining reservations the CPN acted positively, and

agreed to be involved in questionnaire dvelopment. Two elements characterized this phase: development and refinement of survey questionnaire, and
discussions with staff to encourage their involvement. In pursuit of the latter,
the senior CPN initially discussed the project with his team without my
presence, designed to minimize antagonism and allow genuine airing of
views. There were fewer difficulties with the social work team, perhaps
because the researcher was a social worker himself (and hence to be trusted!)
This was followed by a general meeting of both teams, at the end of which
they broadly agreed to go to the next, pilot, stage.

Parallel with this, meetings occurred involving the senior social worker,
senior CPN, another CPN and the researcher (the project research group)
with three purposes: to explain and negotiate the overall research aim and
design, to refine the forms and to engage the interest of the workers at the
centre in the project. The issue of agendas is important here (Weiss, 1972):
the senior CPN in particular wished for information about the work of the
centre as a whole, which he hoped would help justify their work. My main
interest was specifically the work of CPNs and social workers, which was of
secondary interest to him. Fortunately it was possible to undertake both tasks
so there was no conflict of aims. The development of the questionnaire is
discussed below. However, for practical reasons it was important to make
the format as brief as possible consistent with comprehensive cover of issues.
Preliminary trials of the workers' questionnaire were carried out by three
workers who used them over a number of days while on duty, and who
made comments on their practicality. The more extensive pilot is discussed
below.

The Survey

The workers' conduct of cases was researched through a survey of cases
referred. This approach was taken for two main reasons. The primary purpose was to compare the work of CPNs and social workers; the object, then,
was to produce data lending themselves to comparison. Marsh (1982, p. 6)
has commented that surveys are characterized by systematic measures made
over a series of cases, the consistent variables of which are analyzed to see if
they show any patterns, and that the subject matter is social (*cf.* Fowler,
1988). One of the principle advantages of structured questionnaires is that
they provide results which can then be compared with other sources, i.e.
asking the same question to different groups affords the opportunity of
conveniently assessing perspectives of different cohorts over a variety of
issues. Second, such an approach was practical. The examination of about
400 cases imposes certain limitations upon the researcher — particularly
where there is only one — and the survey provided a realistic means for
gathering data. Phillips (1983) suggests that, as a broad guide, where knowledge is thin, small scale qualitative research is probably more fruitful. For

large samples, seeking to establish generalizations, quantitative data are easier to manage. Third, related to the previous point, the data were collected through self administered questionnaires rather than by interview. This was again connected with the practical issue of collecting large amounts of data, which could be consistently collected through a structured questionnaire even when self administered.

Similar survey techniques have been widely used in social work (Goldberg and Wharburton, 1979; Hadley and McGrath, 1984; Howe, 1986; Fisher *et al.*, 1984) and also with CPNs (Sladden, 1979). In this respect we were helped by the experience of previous researchers: the case review questionnaire (CRQ) developed by Goldberg and Wharburton (1979) has been widely used in social work research. However, it was more complex for us for three reasons: it was a social work instrument, not *necessarily* appropriate for CPNs; it was being used in a mental health setting, for which it was not necessarily appropriate; and it contained no detailed reference to mental disorder. Instead, however, of developing an entirely new questionnaire, it was decided to amend that of Goldberg and Wharburton. This had certain advantages: it had been successfully used in a number of studies, it was highly effective in collecting large quantities of data, and it provided a means for collecting data in three monthly stages, facilitating accurate collection. If, furthermore, there was extensive role overlap, as suggested by some CPNs, this instrument would appear relevant to CPNs.

Nonetheless, it did require amendments to be relevant to our study. The development of our questionnaire was based on two key elements: an understanding of the way in which both CPNs and social workers defined their 'professional world' (Chapter 2) and a constant refining of the form in the pre-research phase through meetings between the researcher, CPNs and social workers. The work involved, therefore, in analyzing the theoretical foundations of social work and CPNs, was not simply to compare theory bases, but to provide foundations upon which a research instrument relevant to both professions could be developed. It was important that the instrument was understandable to *both* groups if comparison was to be achieved. It also ensured that results would be relevant to the wider professional audience of CPNs and social workers, rather than being over-concerned with parochial issues. The research instrument is produced in Appendix 2 to this volume. Its connection with the framework for analysis is reasonably clear. Hence, the phenomena with which they were concerned were defined as problems, and divided into three: mental health, social and physical health. Clients were defined in terms of the primary problem which could be any one of the three problem areas and gave expression to the fact that clients were not necessarily primarily defined by mental illness. Causes were identified and classified, context of intervention defined the 'level' at which intervention took place, forms of intervention were classified by role, and change measured through workers' perceptions.

However, definitions also needed to make sense within the everyday working of the service. This was part of the task of the project research group. A number of meetings took place through which the questionnaire was refined, followed by a piloting period of two months during which the workers became acquainted with the forms and final amendments could be made through their use in practice. Each worker was given detailed instructions to be used when completing forms. At the outset reservations, or even outright hostility, of three types, were expressed: a fear of overburdening already busy workers by the demands of research, a dislike of filling in forms, and a fear — not expressed to the researcher but known to the seniors — of the implications of evaluation. Attitudes did change. Acquaintance with, and routine use of the forms reduced anxiety, and trust grew as workers became better acquainted with the researcher, who was gradually transformed from 'outsider' to 'insider'. A significant issue was the care with which the questionnaires were completed. Here the preliminary work of engaging their support was important. Harassed workers may have given them cursory attention, or guessed at some (e.g. demographic) information. Observation by the researcher suggested that they were generally completed with great care: for example, where joint work was undertaken, although one person would complete the form, this would be done with discussion and agreement with the other worker (as indeed, instructions required). The forms were, furthermore, individually checked by both the senior CPN and researcher after completion, and incomplete forms (which were rare) were returned for completion. Only after this were they prepared for processing. However, it should be said that there may have been some variation in the care with which forms were completed, a problem common to all approaches of this sort. Finally, where cases were allocated, three monthly assessments were completed. This helped maximize accuracy, particularly where cases were open for some time (e.g. over a year) with the danger of post hoc memory problems.

Although amendments to the Goldberg and Wharburton questionnaire occurred elsewhere, the most notable was the addition of the classification of mental illness. Other studies have used varying approaches, including screening instruments (Goldberg, 1972), standardized research instruments (Wing et al., 1974), diagnosis by psychiatrist or case register data (Wooff, 1987). Fisher et al. (1984) felt precise psychiatric disorder was insufficiently understood by area social workers to be used in research, and had broad concepts of impairment of mental state and social functioning. Although it was equally important to use language meaningful to workers, psychiatric terminology was regularly used by these social workers and CPNs based in a specialist psychiatric setting. All but one social worker was approved, all the CPNs were RMN trained, and all of both groups had a number of years post qualifying experience. Additionally these workers were seen as specialists by outside professionals such as GPs, nurses and district social workers as well as psychiatrists. They were frequently referred clients for psychiatric assessment and a great deal of trust was placed in them in this respect by these professionals. The use of psychiatric terminology therefore appeared appropriate as an aspect of their definitions of clients. The classifications of mental disorder were developed with the project team, using categories derived from the Ninth International Classification of Disease (WHO, 1977). This enabled us to identify those disorders most frequently confronted at the centre, and to use terminology meaningful to the workers. This had implications for drug and alcohol abuse. While other disorders were distinctively in neurotic or psychotic groups, alcohol and drug abuse in our classification contained both psychotic and neurotic elements (291 alcoholic psychosis, 303 alcohol dependence syndrome; 292 drug psychoses and 304 drug dependence). This was because workers felt these categories best represented these problems and that further distinctions would unnecessarily complicate the forms. As with other categories instructions given to workers gave definitions of each disorder.

The distinction between definite and borderline cases was largely one of severity. It is a distinction common in standardized instruments (Brown and Harris, 1978; Goldberg and Huxley, 1980). although of course in this case it involved the judgment of individual professionals rather than standardized responses. To be rated definite, the person would have to be sufficiently disturbed that a psychiatrist would not be surprised to see them in out patients (or hospitalized) and likely to benefit from psychiatric treatment. Borderline cases had symptoms of a disorder, but their symptoms were not sufficient in number or severity to be rated cases. (Brown and Harris, 1978). This, of course, involved judgment. Goldberg and Huxley (1980) note the cut off point between cases and non cases is arbitrary, though attempting to reflect current standards and Clare (1980) points out there is no hard and fast distinction between mental illness and health, but there is a continuum, involving a grey area. The borderline category attempted to incorporate this 'grey' element.

Client Interviews

Client perspectives have become recognized as an increasingly important element of service evaluation in recent years (Fisher, 1983; Munton, 1990). It has, however, played a relatively small part in mental health research. This reflects an ideology where little importance is attached to the mentally ill person's view, and where the nature and change in these peoples' problems can be defined only by trained experts — encapsulated in 'cognitive superiority' (Sheppard, 1990). Interviewing clients about intervention is fraught with difficulty. It involves the meeting of (at least) three worlds: that of the client, the worker and researcher. Both conducting interviews and interpreting results should be undertaken with great care. However, it has the great advantage of providing a perspective other than that of the worker on the phenomena under study. Second, as a result, it alters the power relationship implicit in the reporting of results. Where only the 'voice' of the worker would otherwise be heard, that of the client is heard also.

A number of stages were involved in gaining access to clients. Agency agreement was not initially forthcoming. Seniors initially voiced reservations around issues of confidentiality and distressing the client. However, they did agree to consider it later. This was a reflection of their understandable wariness early in the research process; greater familiarity was necessary to build up trust. Interviewing clients placed them (the agency) in a vulnerable position; they needed to be sure the conduct of the researcher did not place them in a bad light; there was an issue of confidentiality in letting me see clients; and negative views would reflect badly on the agency. The research began, therefore, without the certainty of including client interviews. However, the timing of the project made this ultimately unproblematic, within a few months this was fully supported, well before interviews were to begin.

The clients' permission was also required. A letter was sent to each client chosen, on agency paper and signed by the seniors, requesting an interview. In an attempt to minimize refusal clients were asked to reply only if they did *not* wish to be interviewed (a stamped addressed envelope was included). While, however, this agency introduction was necessary for access it involved a further problem. Although introduced as a polytechnic lecturer, the letter may have created the impression of being an 'insider', rather than independent. Furthermore, there may have been some fear about confidentiality (which, however, was not expressed) although confidentiality was stressed in the letter and emphasized at the beginning of the interview. Such factors may affect responses, creating some reluctance to criticize the service. Cornwell (1984) distinguishes 'public accounts' where interviewees reply in ways designed to be acceptable to others, from 'private accounts' which spring directly from personal experience, and are more likely in a trusting relationship. As with other single interview client studies there was a danger that some responses reflected 'public accounts'. However, it should be noted that many clients did feel able to express criticisms of workers.

Interviews have the advantage, over observation, of not being limited to what the researcher can immediately perceive or experience: respondents are able to provide masses of information about themselves (Ackroyd and Hughes, 1981), although they presuppose that they represent adequate reports of respondent perceptions of their circumstances. Interviews were carried out retrospectively, following intervention completion. Rees and Wallace (1982) have commented on the potential problem of recall, and clients may realign their recollections according to subsequent experience or even mood ('search after meaning') (Brown and Harris, 1978). To counter this, interviews were arranged as soon as possible following intervention ceasing. With brief intervention, letters were sent to clients after the allocation meeting the Monday following intervention. With extended intervention, a letter signed by the worker was sent with brief intervention. The overwhelming majority were interviewed between two and three weeks after seeing the worker; on three occasions interviews were delayed through client unavailability, but occurred within a month. All extended clients were interviewed within a month. Others have commented that interviews represent a 'snapshot' in which, unprepared, they may answer without sufficient thought (Fisher, 1983). However, the letter made clear the intention of the interview, and they thus had time to consider their responses. Indeed many clients appeared to have given prior thought to what to say. Some authors (e.g. Sainsbury *et al.*, 1982) suggest that rather than one single interview, multiple interviews monitoring changes in views should be undertaken during intervention, and others have commented that client expectations change with accumulating experience (Locker and Dunt, 1978).

However, post intervention interviews had clear advantages. Many clients were extremely distressed during intervention. There were serious ethical problems about a researcher intruding into the personal distress of clients for his own purposes. Indeed, in practice, the agency would not have allowed this. Second, we aimed to get an overview by clients of their perceptions of intervention: earlier interviews would provide partial views only. Indeed we sought client perceptions of outcome, which could only be supplied following intervention. In both cases, this facilitated comparison with workers' views. Finally, the entirely practical issue of resources meant that one researcher could only feasibly interview a large number of clients once: appropriately at intervention completion.

Choosing Clients

We attempted to obtain groups of clients broadly representative of the total CPN and social work client groups in order to facilitate comparative analysis. An initial problem is who, exactly, *is* the client (Phillips, 1983)? Where, for example a family is involved, should not the whole family be interviewed (Sainsbury, 1975)? Some studies have been criticized for inconsistent identification of clients. In this case the client was defined by the worker as the person with whom they were primarily involved. Of course, the problem can involve more than one person: a depressed man supported by his wife may well place some burden upon her, or a woman's depression may arise from poor marital relations. Although, then, we used consistent criteria, it may be that some, upon whom the impact of intervention was felt, are silent in this account. Interviews were, with three exceptions located in clients' own homes. Two CPN clients were interviewed at the centre, and one social work client at their workplace.

The choice of clients was based on a stratified sample of those attending the centre. The client groups were first divided into two: those receiving brief and those receiving extended intervention reflecting the administrative division in the agency. The emphasis also generally differed. Brief intervention normally involved one or two interviews over a few days designed to manage immediate problems or crises, or referral to other agencies. Extended intervention assumed the need to examine and work on problems over time. The clients might be expected to experience these differently, with greater demonstrated commitment and relationship development possible with extended work. A further division was that between CPN and social work clients, with extended intervention, and CPN, social work and joint (CPN and social work) clients with brief work. Given the focus on CPNs and social workers, all interviews involving doctors were excluded. Certain brief clients were also excluded: those assessed for compulsory admission and those hospitalized informally. The clients would not generally be fit for interview.

Altogether thirty-nine brief and thirty-eight extended clients, equally divided by professional group, were interviewed. Representativeness presented problems: clients may refuse, or for other reasons (e.g. moving house) be unavailable. Access is often not obtained with a high proportion of clients (Corney, 1981; Fisher *et al.*, 1984). Because of likely refusals, detailed stratification was considered unwise. Primary problem was chosen to stratify clients, since this was the main means by which we 'defined' clients. The division was broad: into those defined as mental health and social problem cases. These were worker definitions; it was unknown beforehand if clients agreed to them. The clients interviewed reflected the proportion of all cases seen by each profession falling into each category. Hence, we had brief and extended; professional group, and case definition as bases for choice. Excluding those assessed for compulsory admission and those hospitalized informally, brief clients seen by each of the professional groups were as follows: social workers saw twelve mental health cases (39 per cent) and nineteen social problem cases; CPNs saw twenty four mental health cases (57 per cent) and eighteen social problem cases; joint workers saw thirty-four mental health cases (39 per cent) and fifty-four social problem cases. Those interviewed (see table 7.2) closely reflected those proportions. However, while timing of interviews made possible a reflection of clients receiving brief intervention (since our study of this ended before client interviews) extended intervention was more complex, since referrals beyond April were included in the extended work study. Instead, we interviewed clients reflecting the proportions referred by April allocated for extended work. The differences between April and study completion are as follows.

	Social Work		CPN	
	Mental Health	*Social*	*Mental Health*	*Social*
April	7 (28 %)	18 (72 %)	10 (59 %)	7 (41 %)
Completion	16 (19 %)	68 (81 %)	33 (56 %)	26 (44 %)

Of CPN clients, 58 per cent of those interviewed (eleven) were mental health cases, close to completion figures, although 74 per cent (fourteen) of social work clients interviewed were social problem cases, a rather wider gap. Additionally worth noting is that extended clients (six CPN and ten social work) were unavailable or refused, as were brief clients (fifteen CPN, thirteen social work and seventeen joint). Where a client refused or was unavailable, we simply chose the next client available who otherwise fitted our criteria. The reasons for this difference between brief and extended clients are a matter for conjecture. Brief clients may have identified less with the service, some whose crisis had passed may have wished to forget the experience, while others may still have felt it and not been up to the interview.

Extended clients interviewed were the subjects of consecutively closed cases, the order of which the researcher had no influence over. However, those closed in a relatively short period (e.g. under three months) would frequently be included, whereas longer term cases, such as those lasting to the end of the study, would not. There was, then, a tendency to favour cases of short-medium duration. Interviews with brief clients occurred after the main day-to-day survey was completed instead. The first client referred each day who only received brief work, and who fitted other criteria, was selected. Although again the researcher could not influence choice of client, it is unknown whether being 'first client' differentiated them from other clients.

Qualitative and Quantitative Elements

One concern, expressed by Rees and Wallace (1982) is that data collected reflects researchers' not clients' concerns: for clients the issues examined in research may not be those they considered most important. Ethnographers emphasize the need to examine subjects' perceptions and frame of reference (Hammersley and Atkinson, 1983). However, it seems reasonable also to examine clients' views of matters considered important by professionals, a process evident (though not explicit) in other studies (Paykel and Griffiths, 1983; Corney, 1981). Our approach, as with the main survey, emphasized examining clients' views through a framework (Chapter 6) drawing on profession defined practice foundations.

Both quantitative and qualitative methods were used, as advocated by Locker and Dunt (1978). Approaches using fully structured questionnaires have been used elsewhere (Sainsbury *et al*, 1982; Corney, 1981; Paykel and Griffiths, 1983). The structured questionnaires were designed to provide categories exactly comparable with workers' questionnaires. This did present some problems. The questionnaire was piloted with the first ten clients interviewed. Clients had some difficulty with mental disorder, involving technical terms and hence less accessible to clients than social problem categories. Some clients were bemused by terms like schizophrenia, and their interpretation of terms like depression or anxiety could reflect lay rather than clinical definitions. However, given the subject matter — mental health — it appeared inappropriate to leave it out. Further, one aspect of intervention may be for workers to communicate and explain their view of client problems. Finally, self perceptions could be compared with those of workers. However, data on mental health should be treated with care. Attempts have been made to take this into account in the text. Other areas of the text provided few difficulties for clients. Where they were unclear the researcher gave some explanation, but left the decision about whether it was appropriate in their case to the client.

Silverman (1985), as noted earlier, has commented that it is insufficient to provide impressionistic or anecdotal evidence based on qualitative methods. Simple counting techniques significantly advance the accuracy of these methods. Further, it considerably facilitates comparative analysis. Open ended questions can produce a mass of different words, concerns and meanings (Stacey, 1969). Classification and counting can help manage this. Clients were asked about workers' intervention using a semi-structured open ended approach. Answers were subject to content analysis, which examined client identification of interpersonal skills, deficiencies in that area, and the difference that the non-involvement of the worker would have made. The skills were identified using the framework of profession defined practice foundations (Chapter 6). Clients' replies were recorded and transcribed using audio tapes (Hammersley and Atkinson, 1983). Weber (1985) comments that content analysis involves classifying words, phrases or other units of text into categories which have common meanings or similar connotations. To achieve this full transcriptions of comments were necessary. However, the results of content analysis were not simply reproduced statistically. Presentation of client accounts was also undertaken; this aimed to give a sense of the way clients presented their views. This provided illustrations of the way clients discussed workers' skills, and also helped show the different ways in which skills were described. Hence the use of qualitative methods helped complement quantitative methods.

Research Questionnaires

Psychiatric Advisory Service: Case Review Questionnaire

CLIENT NUMBER: ☐☐☐
(1–3)

SECTION 1: SOCIAL AND DEMOGRAPHIC INFORMATION.

1. AGE: 19 or under ☐ 20–44 ☐ 45–64 ☐   65 or above ☐   (4)
             1   2   3   4

2. SEX: Male ☐   Female ☐   (5)
              1   2

3. MARITAL STATUS: Single .... ☐ 1   Widowed ...... ☐ 4
                    Cohabiting ..... ☐ 2   Divorced .... ☐ 5   (6)
                    Married .... ☐ 3   Separated ..... ☐ 6

4. HOUSING CONDITION: Owner occupied ..... ☐ 1   Lodger/landlady .... ☐ 4
                       Private rented .... ☐ 2   Hostel .... ☐ 5   (7)
                       Council .... ☐ 3   No fixed abode .... ☐ 6

5. NUMBER OF CHILDREN IN THE HOUSE AGED 15 OR UNDER:

	1	2	3	4	5	6	7	8	
Age 0–4 years	☐	☐	☐	☐	☐	☐	☐	☐	(8)
Age 5–15 years	☐	☐	☐	☐	☐	☐	☐	☐	(9)

6. OCCUPATION OF CLIENT:
   Employment .... (state)
   Unemployed .... ☐
   Housewife .... ☐

7. OCCUPATION OF PARTNER:
   Employment .... (state)
   Unemployed .... ☐
   Housewife .... ☐

8. PLACE OF WORK, INDUSTRY OR BUSINESS: This refers to the main concerns or 'product' of their place of work, e.g. advertising agency, engineering firm, agriculture, housing department, school/education, building contractors, forestry etc.

Client ....
Partner ....

☐ (10)
☐ (11)
Socioeconomic group. LEAVE THESE BOXES (10 and 11) BLANK.

9. PART TIME WORK: If employed, does client or partner work full time or part time?

Client: full time ☐ 1 (12)
           part time ☐ 2

Partner: full time ☐ 1 (13)
            part time ☐ 2

10. DO THEY RECEIVE STATE BENEFIT? Yes.... ☐ 1 (14)
                                     No ..... ☐ 2

Is this: Family income supplement   ☐ YES 1 ☐ NO 2 (15)
         Unemployment/Supplementary Benefit ☐ YES 1 ☐ NO 2 (16)
         Sickness/Invalidity Benefit   ☐ YES 1 ☐ NO 2 (17)
         Other   ☐ YES 1 ☐ NO 2 (18)

11. IF CLIENT NOT BORN IN BRITAIN, COUNTRY OF BIRTH: ....

SECTION 2: REFERRAL INFORMATION. To be filled in on duty, or if not possible, at first subsequent interview.

1. REFERRAL STATUS: New Referral .... ☐ 1 (19)
                     Previously known ... ☐ 2

2. REFERRED BY: Please *ring* the appropriate number, corresponding to referrer.

Self ....1 Voluntary services 8   Casualty 15
Relative 2   District Social Worker 9   General Hospital ward 16
Friend/acquaintance ..3   GP. 10   Psychiatric Hospital ward .17
Police 4   CPN. 11   Day hospital 18 (20–21)
Probation 5   District nurse 12   Psychologist 19
DHSS/Housing 6   Health visitor................13   Qualified Psychiatrist 20
Service Welfare 7   Hospital Social Worker .14   Other Hospital doctor 21
                                                                 Other   22
                                                                 (state):
                                                                 ....

3. WAS REFERRAL ADVISORY/SUPPLEMENTARY TO CURRENT PSYCHIATRIC/SOCIAL WORK INTERVENTION?

Current CPN caseload ....☐ 1   Psychiatrist ....☐ 3   Psychologist ....☐ 5
Current Mental Health   District Social Worker/   No current   (22)
Social Work caseload .....☐ 2   Probation ....☐ 4   intervention .....☐ 6

4. MODE OF REFERRAL: letter ....☐ 1   visit to office ....☐ 3 (23)
                      telephone ....☐ 2   other ....☐ 4

5. REQUEST BY REFERRER: Please indicate which of the following categories represents the MAIN activity requested by referrer. *Tick one box only.*

Assessment ....☐ 1
Advice ....☐ 2
Material help ....☐ 3   (24)
Counselling/emotional support ....☐ 4
Medication ....☐ 5
Hospital Admission ....☐ 6

6. MENTAL DISORDER: (a) Indicate which of the following disorders you felt was evident at first interview. Please *indicate only ONE* (i.e. tick only one box). Do not worry if your assessment is only provisional. (b) If referred by a GP or Psychiatrist, indicate *their* diagnosis (*if available at referral*).

	Referring doctor		Yours			Referring doctor		Yours
None	☐	1	☐		Schizophrenia	☐	8	☐
Depression	☐	2	☐		Dementia (senile/			
Anxiety	☐	3	☐		pre-senile)	☐	9	☐
Phobic	☐	4	☐		Alcohol abuse	☐	10	☐
Obsessive/compulsive	☐	5	☐		Drug abuse	☐	11	☐
Personality Disorder	☐	6	☐		Other	☐	12	☐
Mania/manic depressive					(specify):			
Psychosis	☐	7	☐		....			

CODE: Please leave these boxes (25 and 26) blank.
Doctor ......☐☐   (25)
Self ....☐☐   (26)

7. ASSOCIATED SOCIAL AND PHYSICAL HEALTH PROBLEMS: Indicated (a) by referrer in referral and (b) at first interview. Again, it is recognized that your assessment may be provisional at first interview. Please try to *avoid* the unclear box as far as possible: only tick it if you literally have no idea what the problems are.

	Referral		First Interview			Referral		First Interview	
Housing	☐	(27)	☐	(42)	Emotional	☐	(36)	☐	(51)
Financial	☐	(28)	☐	(43)	Delinquency/				
Employment	☐	(29)	☐	(44)	Criminal behaviour	☐	(37)	☐	(52)
Home management	☐	(30)	☐	(45)	Major physical ill				
Marital	☐	(31)	☐	(46)	health/disability	☐	(38)	☐	(53)
Child abuse/neglect	☐	(32)	☐	(47)	Minor physical ill				
Other child care	☐	(33)	☐	(48)	health/disability	☐	(39)	☐	(54)
Loss/separation	☐	(34)	☐	(49)	Unclear	☐	(40)	☐	(55)
Other social					Other				
relations/isolation	☐	(35)	☐	(50)	(state)	☐	(41)	☐	(56)

CASE REVIEW QUESTIONNAIRE
Completion/3 month schedule.

1. INTERVIEWS: How many face to face interviews do you estimate you had with each of the following (please give an exact number).

Client alone ....☐☐   (57–58)
Spouse or family *alone* ....☐☐   (59–60)
Friends/acquaintances alone ....☐☐   (61–62)
Client plus spouse or family ....☐☐   (63–64)
Client plus friends/acquaintances ....☐☐   (65–66)
Group work ....☐☐   (67–68)

2. ACTIVITIES UNDERTAKEN: Please indicate (a) which activities were undertaken and (b) which *ONE* was most effective.

	(a) UNDERTAKEN	(b) MOST EFFECTIVE
Drug treatment	☐ (2)	☐ 1
Mental health section assessment	☐ (3)	☐ 2
Other assessment/exploration	☐ (4)	☐ 3
Information/advice	☐ (5)	☐ 4
Discussing future options	☐ (6)	☐ 5
Monitoring	☐ (7)	☐ 6 (13–14)
Education in social skills	☐ (8)	☐ 7
Psychodynamic work	☐ (9)	☐ 8
Ventilation/emotional support/sustain	☐ (10)	☐ 9
Advocacy on behalf of client	☐ (11)	☐ 10
Mobilizing resources (e.g. family aide, residential facilities etc.)	☐ (12)	☐ 11

3. MENTAL DISORDER: (a) Please indicate which mental disorder most accurately depicted the client's/patient's mental state. Please indicate only *ONE*. (b) Please indicate if it *either* improved *or* was completely resolved *or* deteriorated. If no change occurred in their mental condition, leave boxes on outcome blank.

	Present 1	OUTCOME Improved 2	Resolved 3	Deteriorated 4	
None	☐	☐	☐	☐	(15)
Depression	☐	☐	☐	☐	(16)
Anxiety	☐	☐	☐	☐	(17)
Phobic	☐	☐	☐	☐	(18)
Obsessive/compulsive behaviour	☐	☐	☐	☐	(19)
Personality disorder	☐	☐	☐	☐	(20)
Mania/manic depressive psychosis.	☐	☐	☐	☐	(21)
Schizophrenia	☐	☐	☐	☐	(22)
Dementia (senile/pre-senile)	☐	☐	☐	☐	(23)
Alcohol abuse	☐	☐	☐	☐	(24)
Drug abuse	☐	☐	☐	☐	(25)
Other (specify)	☐	☐	☐	☐	(26)

4. PSYCHIATRIC STATE: Which of the following most accurately depicts their psychiatric state?

Definite psychiatric disorder ☐ 1.
Borderline psychiatric disorder ☐ 2. (27)
Definitely not psychiatric disorder ☐ 3.

5. SOCIAL AND PHYSICAL ILL HEALTH PROBLEMS: Please indicate, by *ringing* the appropriate number relating to the relevant problems (a) what you considered were the client's problems, (b) which of these you considered *severe* problems, (c) which problems were *tackled* in interview with the client, (d) which were tackled *indirectly* through work with, or referral to, an outside agency/professional (if any problems *not* tackled do not fill in column (c) and (d) in relation to that *particular* problem, (e) Indicate which problems *improved* (mildly or markedly) during intervention, (f) indicate which problems *deteriorated* during intervention. If the situation stayed the same (i.e. no improvement or deterioration) in relation to a particular problem, do not fill in column (e) and (f) in relation to that *particular* problem.

			TACKLED		OUTCOME				
(a)	(b)	(c) in interview	(d) indirectly	(e) Improved mild marked		(f) Deteriorated mild marked			
	Present	Severe							
Housing ....(2)	(16)	(30)	(44)	3	4	5	6	(58)
Financial ....(3)	(17)	(31)	(45)	3	4	5	6	(59)
Employment ....(4)	(18)	(32)	(46)	3	4	5	6	(60)
Home management .(5)	(19)	(33)	(47)	3	4	5	6	(61)
Marital ....(6)	(20)	(34)	(48)	3	4	5	6	(62)
Child abuse/neglect .(7)	(21)	(35)	(49)	3	4	5	6	(63)
Other child care ....(8)	(22)	(36)	(50)	3	4	5	6	(64)
Loss/separation ....(9)	(23)	(37)	(51)	3	4	5	6	(65)
Other social relations/ isolation ....(10)	(24)	(38)	(52)	3	4	5	6	(66)
Emotional ....(11)	(25)	(39)	(53)	3	4	5	6	(67)
Delinquency/criminal behaviour................(12)	(26)	(40)	(54)	3	4	5	6	(68)
Major physical ill health/disability ......(13)	(27)	(41)	(55)	3	4	5	6	(69)
Minor physical ill health/disability ......(14)	(28)	(42)	(56)	3	4	5	6	(70)
Other (specify)	(15)	(29)	(43)	(57)	3	4	5	6	(71)

FOR CODING ONLY: PAS workers IGNORE numbers (58)–(71)

6. CAUSE: Which of the following do you consider to have been the *main* factor precipitating the problem? (please tick *ONE* box only).

Sudden practical/health event impacting on client (e.g. learning of a relative's cancer, being burgled, receiving an unexpectedly heavy bill the client cannot afford, loss of job) ....☐ 1

Sudden relationship event (e.g. loss/bereavement of loved one, losing friends through moving house, discovering partner is unfaithful) ....☐ 2

Behaviour/attitude of client ....☐ 3

Behaviour/attitude of relatives/acquaintances/friends ....☐ 4   (2)

Combined behaviour/attitude of client/relatives/acquaintances ....☐ 5

Persistent material/practical problems..☐ 6

Persistent ill health/disability problems in client/relatives ....☐ 7

Psychophysiological problems (ie clients/patients whose problems appear to arise from organic/biochemical bodily disorders) ....☐ 8

Failure to take prescribed medication ....☐ 9

7. OUTSIDE AGENCIES CONTACTED: Please estimate the number of contacts you made with each of the following agencies (including letter, telephone, face to face).

DHSS .... ☐☐	(3–4)
Housing department .... ☐☐	(5–6)
Social Service personnel/resources .. ☐☐	(7–8)
Consultant Psychiatrist .... ☐☐	(9–10)
GP .... ☐☐	(11–12)
Other health personnel/resources .... ☐☐	(13–14)
Drug/alcohol unit .... ☐☐	(15–16)
Police/probation/solicitor .... ☐☐	(17–18)
Voluntary .... ☐☐	(19–20)
Other (specify) .... ☐☐	(21–22)

8. REFERRAL ON: Was the client/patient referred on to any of the following for intervention or treatment?

Psychiatric 'in-patient'	☐	(23)	Social worker/Social Services	☐	(28)
Psychiatric 'out-patient'	☐	(24)	General Practitioner	☐	(29)
CPN (rehabilitation/elderly)	☐	(25)	Service Welfare	☐	(30)
CPN (general psychiatry)	☐	(26)	Drug/alcohol unit	☐	(31)
Psychologist	☐	(27)	Voluntary organization	☐	(32)
			Other (state)	☐	(33)

9. LENGTH OF INTERVENTION: In days if less than a week, in weeks if less than a month, or in months.

Months ☐☐ (34–35)   Weeks ☐☐ (36–37)   Days ☐☐ (38–39)

10. MAIN OR SOLE PAS WORKER INVOLVED:

Other PAS workers involved:

☐☐ 40–41)
(42–43)   (44–45)
☐☐   ☐☐

11. WHERE PATIENT/CLIENT REFERRED ON TO OUTSIDE PROFESSIONALS FOR INTERVENTION OR TREATMENT: i.e. when indicated in question 8: did you give the professional advice on any of the following in relation to the client/patient (please tick appropriate box).

Psychiatric condition/diagnosis	☐	(46)	Emotional/relationship problems	☐	(49)
Physical health/ill health	☐	(47)	Case management techniques	☐	(50)
Practical/financial problems	☐	(48)	None of these	☐	(51)

12. PRIMARY PROBLEM: Which of the following psychiatric/social problems would you consider to be the primary problem of the client (Ring one number only).

Depression	1	Housing	12
Anxiety	2	Financial	13
Phobic	3	Employment	14
Obsessive/compulsive	4	Home management	15
Personality disorder	5	Marital	16
Mania/manic depressive	6	Child abuse/neglect	17
Schizophrenia	7	Other child care	18
Dementia (senile/pre-		Loss/separation	19
senile	8	Other social relations/	
Alcohol abuse	9	isolation	20
Drug abuse	10	Emotional	21
Other psychiatric		Delinquency/criminal	
(specify):		behaviour	22
		Major Physical ill health	
	11	or disability	23
		Major physical ill health	
		or disability	24
		Other social/health	
		(specify):	25

☐☐ (52–53)

13. CASELOAD ALLOCATION: What was the status of the case?

	Brief only	☐	1
Caseload	Short Term	☐	2
	Long Term	☐	3 (54)
	Medical	☐	4
	Allocated/Not seen	☐	5

14. REASON FOR CASE CLOSURE:

☐☐ (55–56)

Client Interview Questionnaire

1. SOCIAL AND PHYSICAL ILL HEALTH PROBLEMS: Looking back, what do you think, from the following list, were your problems?
Which problems did the worker think you had? Which were tackled by/with the worker?
Did their intervention help ease or resolve the problems?

	Problem presence			Intervention Effect				
				Improved		Deteriorated		
	Client's View	Of Worker's View	Tackled	Mild	Marked	Mild	Marked	
Housing	(2)	(3)	(4)	3	4	5	6	(5)
Financial	(6)	(7)	(8)	3	4	5	6	(9)
Employment	(10)	(11)	(12)	3	4	5	6	(13)
Home management	(14)	(15)	(16)	3	4	5	6	(17)
Marital	(18)	(19)	(20)	3	4	5	6	(21)
Child abuse/neglect	(22)	(23)	(24)	3	4	5	6	(25)
Other child care	(26)	(27)	(28)	3	4	5	6	(29)
Loss/separation	(30)	(31)	(32)	3	4	5	6	(33)
Other social relations/ isolation	(34)	(35)	(36)	3	4	5	6	(37)
Emotional	(38)	(39)	(40)	3	4	5	6	(41)
Delinquency/criminal behaviour	(42)	(43)	(44)	3	4	5	6	(45)
Major physical ill health/disability	(46)	(47)	(48)	3	4	5	6	(49)
Minor physical ill health/disability	(50)	(51)	(52)	3	4	5	6	(53)
Other (specify)	(54)	(55)	(56)	3	4	5	6	(57)

2. PSYCHIATRIC PROBLEMS: Looking back, do you think you had any of the following problems? Which problems did the worker think you had?

	Client's view		Of Worker's view		
None	☐	1	☐	1	
Depression	☐	2	☐	2	
Anxiety	☐	3	☐	3	
Phobic	☐	4	☐	4	
Obsessive/compulsive	☐	5	☐	5	
Personality disorder	☐	6	☐	6	
Mania/manic depressive Psychosis	☐	7	☐	7	
Schizophrenia	☐	8	☐	8	
Dementia	☐	9	☐	9	
Alcohol abuse	☐	10	☐	10	
Drug abuse	☐	11	☐	11	
Other (specify)	☐	12	☐	12	

Client's view (58–59) Of Worker's view (60–61)

5a. OUTCOME.
improved   1
resolved   2   (62)
deteriorated 3

5b. PRIMARY
PROBLEM.
(social/psychiatric)

☐☐
(63–64)

3. LENGTH OF INVOLVEMENT: How long was the worker involved with you? (in days if less than a week, in weeks if less than a month, or in months).

Months ☐☐ (2–3)   Weeks ☐☐ (4–5)   Days ☐ (6)

How many interviews did you have with the worker? ☐☐ (7–8)

Did you think the amount of time they were involved with you was

Too long .... ☐   1
About right .... ☐   2   (9)
Too short .... ☐   3

If it was too long or too short why do you think this was so?

☐☐ (10–11)

Did you think the number of interviews you had with the worker was

Too many .... ☐   1
About right .... ☐   2   (12)
Too few .... ☐   3

If there were too many or too few, why do you think this was so?

☐☐ (13–14)

4. FOCUS FOR INTERVENTION: (i) Who/what was the main focus for intervention (if an outside agency, indicate which of the other categories—if any—was the main focus involving people) (ii) Did you agree with the worker that this should be the main focus (iii) if you disagreed, which should have been the main focus?

	Main Focus		Focus Agreed		Appropriate Focus (if disagreed)	
Client	☐ 1		☐ 1		☐ 1	
Spouse or family alone	☐ 2		☐ 2		☐ 2	
Friends/acquaintances alone	☐ 3		☐ 3		☐ 3	
Client plus spouse or family	☐ 4	(15)	☐ 4	(16)	☐ 4	(17)
Client plus friends/acquaintances ...	☐ 5		☐ 5		☐ 5	
Group work	☐ 6		☐ 6		☐ 6	
Outside Agencies	☐ 7		☐ 7		☐ 7	

5. ACTIVITIES UNDERTAKEN AND THEIR EFFECTIVENESS: (i) Which of the following activities was undertaken by your worker(s) to help with your problems (ii) Which ONE was the most effective in helping/resolving your problems (ii) Would any alternative activities have been more effective?

	Activities undertaken	most effective activity	(more effective) Alternative activities
Drug treatment	☐ (18)	☐ 1	☐ (19)
Assessment/exploration of problem	☐ (20)	☐ 2	☐ (21)
Giving client information and advice	☐ (22)	☐ 3	☐ (23)
Discussing future options	☐ (24)	☐ 4	☐ (25)
Keeping an eye on the situation	☐ (26)	☐ 5	☐ (27)
Helping client perform social tasks better (education in social skills	☐ (28)	☐ 6	☐ (29)
Psychodynamic work (helping the client understand their own feelings/actions better) ...	☐ (30)	☐ 7	☐ (31)

Giving client emotional
support/opportunity to
ventilate their feelings .... ☐ (32)   ☐ 8   ☐ (33)
Advocacy on clients behalf to
outside agency .... ☐ (34)   ☐ 9   ☐ (35)
Mobilising resources for
practical help (e.g. family aide
residential facilities) .... ☐ (36)   ☐ 10   ☐ (37)

☐☐ (38–39)

6. CAUSE: Which of the following was the *main* cause of your problems? What do you think
the social worker/CPN thought was the main cause?

	Your view		Worker's view (as you perceive)	
Sudden practical/health event	☐ 1		☐ 1	
Sudden relationship event	☐ 2		☐ 2	
Behaviour/attitude of the client	☐ 3		☐ 3	
Behaviour/attitude of relatives/friends etc. ...	☐ 4		☐ 4	
Combined behaviour/attitude of client relatives/friends/acquaintances	☐ 5	(40–41)	☐ 5	(42–43)
Persistent material/practical problems	☐ 6		☐ 6	
Persistent ill health/disability problems in client/relatives	☐ 7		☐ 7	
Psychophysiological problems	☐ 8		☐ 8	
Failure to take prescribed medication	☐ 9		☐ 9	
Not Certain			☐ 10	

7. PERSONAL RESPONSIBILITY FOR PROBLEMS: Did you consider the development of
the/your problems to have been largely out of your control (i.e. that there was really
nothing you could have done which would have prevented its occurrence, and that,
therefore, you could not be made responsible for it).

Yes   ☐   1
                            (44)
No   ☐   2

8. CLIENT PARTICIPATION IN DEFINING/RESOLVING PROBLEMS.

a) Defining client's problems; during intervention, who would you say was responsible for
identifying/defining the problems and difficulties to be tackled?

	1 Mainly/entirely worker	2 Equal responsibility	3 Mainly/entirely client	
Practical/financial	☐	☐	☐	(45)
Child care/familial	☐	☐	☐	(46)
Other social network/relations	☐	☐	☐	(47)
Personal functioning (including social skills/confidence/role performance)	☐	☐	☐	(48)
Ill health	☐	☐	☐	(49)

b) Planning/directiveness of worker: who decided what should be done to tackle the
problems identified in each of the following problem areas?

	1 Mainly/entirely worker	2 Equal responsibility	3 Mainly/entirely client	
Practical/financial	☐	☐	☐	(50)
Child care/familial	☐	☐	☐	(51)
Personal functioning	☐	☐	☐	(52)
Social relation/network	☐	☐	☐	(53)
Ill health	☐	☐	☐	(54)

c) Responsibility for action: Who actually took responsibility for taking action to tackle problems? (e.g. financial problems may be tackled by the client going to DHSS to sort it out, or by the worker doing it himself; the worker may speak to a relative/friend to change their behaviour/attitudes or you may do so after appropriate discussion with the worker; or you may both work on these problems).

	1 Mainly/entirely worker	2 Equal responsibility	3 Mainly/entirely client	
Practical/financial	☐	☐	☐	(55)
Child care/familial	☐	☐	☐	(56)
Personal functioning	☐	☐	☐	(57)
Social relations/network	☐	☐	☐	(58)
Ill health	☐	☐	☐	(59)

d) Openness of worker: Did you feel the worker was open with you in saying what they were thinking and doing in relation to the following problems.

	Open 1	Not open 2	Not relevant 3	
Practical/financial	☐	☐	☐	(60)
Child care/familial	☐	☐	☐	(61)
Personal functioning	☐	☐	☐	(62)
Social relations/network	☐	☐	☐	(63)
Ill health	☐	☐	☐	(64)

9. CLIENT SATISFACTION.

very satisfied	1	
quite satisfied	2	
neither satisfied/ dissatisfied	3	(65)
quite dissatisfied	4	
very dissatisfied	5	

Bibliography

ACKROYD, S. and HUGHES, J. (1981) *Data Collection in Context*, London, Longman.

AIRDOOS, N. (1985) 'Interpersonal skills: Building blocks for a core component in the nursing curriculum', in ALTSCHUL, A. (Ed.) *Psychiatric Nursing*, Edinburgh, Churchill Livingstone.

ALLOY, L.B. (1988) *Cognitive Processes in Depression*, London, The Guilford Press.

ALTSCHUL, A. (1972) *Patient-Nurse Interaction*. London, Churchill Livingstone.

ALTSCHUL, A. (1978) *Psychiatric Nursing*, London, Balliere-Tindall.

ANDERSON, J. (1988) *Foundations of Social Work Practice*, New York, Springer.

ATKINSON, P. (1977) 'The reproduction of professional knowledge', in DINGWALL, R., HEATH, C., REID, M. and STACEY, M. (Eds) *Health Care and Health Knowledge*, London, Croom Helm.

ATKINSON, P. (1983) 'The reproduction of the professional community', in DINGWALL, R. and LEWIS, P. (Eds) *The Sociology of the Professions: Lawyers, Doctors and Others*, London, Macmillan.

AUDIT COMMISSION (1986) *Report of the Audit Commission for Local Authorities in England and Wales*, London, HMSO.

BAILEY, R. and BRAKE, M. (1975) *Radical Social Work*, London, Edward Arnold.

BAKER, F. and SCHULBERG, E. (1967) 'The development of a community mental health ideology scale', *Community Mental Health Journal*, **3**, pp. 216–51.

BANNISTER, P. and KAGAN, C. (1985) 'The Need for Research into Inter-personal Skills in Nursing', in KAGAN, C. (Ed.) *Interpersonal Skills in Nursing*, London, Croom Helm.

BARKER P.J. (1982) *Behavioural Therapy Nursing*, London, Croom Helm.

BARKER, P.J. (1985) *Patient Assessment in Psychiatric Nursing*, London, Croom Helm.

BARRY, P.D. (1984) *Psychosocial Nursing Assessment and Intervention*, London, J.P.L. Lipincott.

BARTLETT, H. (1970) *The Common Base of Social Work Practice*, Washington DC, National Association of Social Workers.

BARTON, W.R. (1959) *Institutional Neurosis*, Bristol, John Wright.

BERNSTEIN, B. (1971) 'On the Classification and Framing of Educational

Knowledge in YOUNG, M.F.D. (Ed.) *Knowledge and Control: New Directions for the Sociology of Education*, London, Collier Macmillan.

BERNSTEIN, B. (1975) *Class Codes and Control. Volume 3. Towards a Theory of Educational Transmissions*, London, Routledge and Kegan Paul.

BESSELL, R. (1971) *Interviewing and Counselling*, London, Batsford.

BIESTEK, F. (1957) *The Casework Relationship*, London, George Allen and Unwin.

BLACK, J., BOWL, R. and BURNS, D. (1983) *Social Work in Context*, London, Tavistock.

BOARDMAN, A. and BOURAS, N. (1988) 'The Mental Health Advice Centre at Lewisham', *Health Trends*, **20**, 2, pp. 59–63.

BOARDMAN, A., BOURAS, N. and CUNDY, J. (1987) *The Mental Health Advice Centre in Lewisham*, Service Usage. Trends 1978–1984, NUPRD, Lewisham.

BOARDMAN, A., BOURAS, N. and WATSON, J. (1986) 'Evaluation of a community mental health centre'. *Acta Psychiatrica* (Belg), **86**, pp. 402–6.

BOTTORFF, J. and D'CRUZ, J. (1984). 'Towards inclusive notion of "patient" and "nurse"', *Journal of Advanced Nursing*, **9**, pp. 549–53.

BOURAS, N. and BROUGH, D. (1982) 'The development of the Mental Health Advice Centre at Lewisham', *Health Trends*, **14**, pp. 66–69.

BOURAS, N. and TUFFNALL, G. (1983) *Mental Health Advice Centre. The Crisis Intervention Team*, Lewisham Health Authority.

BRANDON, D. (1981) *Voices of Experience: Consumer Perspective of Psychiatric Treatment*, London, MIND.

BRIDGE, W. and MCLEOD-CLARK, J. (1986) *Communication in Nursing Care*, London, H. Mandill.

BRISCOE, M., WINNEY, J., CHANDLER, V., MULGREW, K., WILLIMENT, S. and RUSHTON, A. (1983) 'Long term social work in a primary health care setting', *British Journal of Social Work*, **13**, pp. 559–78.

BROOKER, C. (1990) 'A six year follow up study of nurses attending a course in community psychiatric nursing', in BROOKER, C. (Ed.) *Nursing: A Research Perspective*, London, Routledge.

BROOKING, J. (Ed.) (1986) *Psychiatric Nursing Research*, New York, McGraw Hill.

BROWN, G.W., CRAIG, T.K. and HARRIS, T.O. (1985) 'Depression: Distress or Disease?' *British Journal of Psychiatry*, **147**, pp. 612–22.

BROWN, G.W., DAVIDSON, S. and HARRIS, T. (1977) 'Psychiatric Disorder in London and North Uist', *Social Science and Medicine*, **11**, pp. 367–77.

BROWN, G.W. and HARRIS, T.O. (1978) *Social Origins of Depression*, London, Tavistock.

BROWN, R. (1973) 'Feedback in family Interviewing', *Social Work*, **18**, 5, pp. 52–9.

BRYMON, A. (1988) *Quantity and Quality in Social Research*, London, Unwin Hyman.

BUCHER, R. and STRAUSS, A. (1966) 'Professions in Process', *American Journal of Sociology*, **66**, pp. 325–34.

BURGESS, A.W. (1985) *Psychiatric Nursing in the Hospital and Community*, Englewood Cliffs NJ, Prentice Hall.

BURGESS, R. (1984) *In the Field*, London, Allen and Unwin.

BURNARD, P. (1985) *Learning Human Skills*, London, Heinemann.

BURR, J. and ANDREWS, J. (1981) *Nursing the Psychiatric Patient*, Fourth Edition, London, Balliere-Tindall.

BURRELL, G. and MORGAN, G. (1979) *Sociological Paradigms and Organizational Analysis*, London, Heinemann.

BUTLER, A. and PRITCHARD, C. (1983) *Social Work and Mental Illness*, London, Macmillan.

BUTTERWORTH, C. (1984) 'The future training of psychiatric nurses', *Nursing Times*, 25 July, pp. 65–6.

CARPENTER, M. (1977) 'The New Managerialism and Professionalism in Nursing', in STACEY, M. (Ed.) *Health and the Division of Labour*, London, Croom Helm.

CARR, P.J., BUTTERWORTH, C.A. and HODGES, B.E. (1980) *Community Psychiatric Nursing*, London, Churchill Livingstone.

CCETSW (1986) *Paper 19.17 Approved Social Workers: Report of the CCETSW Examinations Board*, London, CCETSW.

CHALLIS, D. and FERLIE, E. (1986) 'Changing patterns of fieldwork organization: The headquarters view'. *British Journal of Social Work*, **16**, pp. 181–202.

CHALLIS, D. and FERLIE, E. (1987) 'Changing patterns of fieldwork organization: II the team leaders' view', *British Journal of Social Work*, **17**, pp. 147–67.

CHAPMAN, C.M. (1985) *Theory of Nursing: Practical Application*, London, Harper and Row.

CHRISMAN, M. and FOWLER, M. (1980) 'The systems change model for nursing practice', in RIEHL, J.P. and ROY, C. (Eds) *Conceptual Models for Nursing Practice*, Second Edition, London, Prentice Hall.

CLARE, A. (1980) *Psychiatry in Dissent*, London, Tavistock.

COCHRANE, R. (1983) *The Social Creation of Mental Illness*, Hong Kong, Longmans.

COHEN, J. and FISHER, M. (1987) 'Recognition of mental health problems by doctors and social workers', *Practice*, **3**, pp. 225–40.

COLLINS, J. and COLLINS, M. (1981) *Achieving Change in Social Work*. London, Heinemann.

COMPTON, B. and GALLOWAY, B. (1979) *Social Work Processes*, Homewood Illinois, The Dorsey Press.

COOPER, B., HARWIN, B., DEPLA, C. and SHEPPARD, M. (1975) 'Mental health in the community: An evaluative study', *Psychological Medicine*, **5**, pp. 372–80.

CORDEN, J. and PRESTON-SHOOT, M. (1987) *Contracts in Social Work*, Aldershot, Gower.

CORMACK, D. (1976) *Psychiatric Nursing Observed*, London, Royal College of Nursing.

CORNEY, R. (1980) 'A comparative study of referrals to a local authority intake team with a general practice attachment scheme', *Social Science and Medicine*, **14**, pp. 675–82.

CORNEY, R. (1981) 'Client Perspectives in a General Practice Attachment', *British Journal of Social Work*, **11**, pp. 159–70.

CORNEY, R. (1984a) *The Effectiveness of Attached Social Workers in the Management of Depressed Female Patients in General Practice*, Cambridge, Cambridge University Press.

CORNEY, R. (1984b) 'The mental and physical health of clients referred to social workers in local authority and a general practice attachment scheme', *Psychological Medicine*, **14**, pp. 137–44.

CORNWELL, J. (1984) *Hard Earned Lives*, London, Tavistock.

COROB, A. (1987) *Working with Depressed Women: A Feminist Approach*, Aldershot, Gower.

CORRIGAN, P. and LEONARD, P. (1978) *Social Work Practice Under Capitalism — A Marxist Approach*, London, Macmillan.

CPNA (1985a) *Clinical Nursing Responsibilities of the Community Psychiatric Nurse*, Bristol, CPNA.

CPNA (1985b) *The 1985 CPNA National Survey Update*, Bristol, CPNA.

CRAIG, T., BOARDMAN, A. and SAYCE, L. (1990) 'Community Mental Health Centres in the United Kingdom', Unpublished, National Unit for Psychiatric Research and Development.

CROWE, R. (1982) 'How nursing and community can benefit from nursing research', *International Journal of Nursing Studies*, **19**, pp. 37–45.

CURNOCK, C. and HARDIKER, P. (1979) *Towards Practice Theory*, London, Routledge and Kegan Paul.

D'ARCY, P. (1984). *Theory and Practice of Psychiatric Care*, London, Hodder and Stoughton.

DARTINGTON, T., NURSE, G. and WILSON, M. (1977) 'Preparing nurses for counselling', *Nursing Mirror*, **44**, pp. 54–5.

DAVEY, P.T. (1984) *Theory and Practice of Psychiatric Care*, London, Hodder and Stoughton.

DAVIES, M. (1974) 'The current state of social work research', *British Journal of Social Work*, **4**, pp. 281–305.

DAVIES, M. (1981) 'Social Work, The State and The University', *British Journal of Social Work*, **11**, pp. 275–88.

DAVIES, M. (1982) 'A Comment on Heart or Head', *Issues in Social Work Education*, **2**, 1, pp. 57–60.

DAVIES, M. (1986) *The Essential Social Worker*, Second Edition, Aldershot, Gower.

DAVIS, A., NEWTON, S. and SMITH, D. (1985) 'Coventry crisis intervention team: The consumers' view' *Social Services Research*, **14**, 1, pp. 7–30.

DAVIS, B. (1986) 'A review of recent research in psychiatric nursing', in BROOKING, J. (Ed.) *Psychiatric Nursing Research*, Chichester, John Wiley and Son.

DAY, P. (1981) *Social Work and Social Control*, London, Tavistock.

DENZIN, N.K. (1978) *The Research Act*, Second Edition, London, McGraw Hill.

DEPARTMENT OF HEALTH (1988) *Health and Personal Social Services Statistics for England: 1988 Edition*, London, HMSO.

DEPARTMENT OF HEALTH (1989) *Caring for People: Community Care in the Next Decade and Beyond*, London, HMSO.

DHSS (1974) *Social Work Support for the Health Service: Report of Working Party* (Ottan Report), London, HMSO.

DHSS (1975a) *Better Services for the Mentally Ill*, London, HMSO.

DHSS (1975b) *Social Work Support for the Health Service: Report of the Working Party*. (Ottan Report), London, HMSO.

DHSS (1978) *Collaboration in Community Care: A Discussion Document*, London, HMSO.

DICK, D. (1985) 'Community Mental Health Centres — Two Models' in

MCAUSLAND, T. (Ed.) *Planning and Monitoring Community Mental Health Centres*, Kings Fund, Unpublished.

ECHLIN, R. (Ed.) (1988) *Community Mental Health Centres/Teams Information Pack*, London, Good Practices in Mental Health.

ENB (1989) *Nursing Care of Mentally Ill People in the Community: Course 812*, London, ENB.

ENGLAND, H. (1986) *Social Work as Art*, London, Allen and Unwin.

EPSTEIN, L. (1985) *Talking and Listening*, St. Louis, Times Mirror/Mosby College Publishing.

FAULKENER, A. (1985) 'The Organizational Context of Interpersonal Skills in Nursing', in KEGAN, C. (Ed.) *Interpersonal Skills in Nursing*, London, Croom Helm.

FERRARD, M. and HUNNYBUN, N. (1964) *The Caseworker's Use of Relationships*, Tavistock, London.

FICHTER, J.H. (1961) *Religion as an Occupation*, South Bend, IN, University of Notre Dame Press.

FISHER, M. (1983) 'The Meaning of Client Satisfaction' in FISHER, M. (Ed.) *Speaking of Clients*, Sheffield, JUSSR, University of Sheffield Press.

FISHER, M., NEWTON, C. and SAINSBURY, E. (1984) *Mental Health Social Work Observed*, London, George Allen and Unwin.

FITZGERALD, R. (1978) 'The classification and recording of social problems', *Social Science and Medicine*, **12**, pp. 255–63.

FLASKERIND, J., HOLLORAM, E. and JANKEN, J. (1979) 'Avoidance and Distancing: A Descriptive View of Nursing', *Nursing Forum*, **18**, p. 158.

FOWLER, F.J. (1988) *Survey Research Methods*, London, Sage.

FREIDSON, E. (1970) *The Profession of Medicine*, New York, Harper and Row.

FRENCH, P. (1983) *Social Skills for Nursing Practice*, London, Croom Helm.

FRYDMAN, M.I. (1981) 'Social support, life events and psychiatric symptoms: A study of direct conditional and interaction effects', *Social Psychiatry*, **16**, pp. 69–78.

GERMAIN, C. and GITTERMAN, A. (1980) *The Life Model of Social Work Practice*, New York.

GIBBONS, J.S., BOW, I., BUTLER, J. and POWELL, J. (1979) 'Clients' reactions to task centred casework: A follow up', *British Journal of Social Work*, **9**, 2, pp. 203–15.

GIBBONS, J.S., BUTLER, I., URWIN, P. and GIBBONS, J.L. (1978) 'Evaluation of a social work service for self poisoning patients', *British Journal of Psychiatry*, **133**, pp. 111–18.

GOFFMAN, E. (1961) *Asylums*, New York, Anchor Books.

GOLDBERG, D. (1972) *The Detection of Psychiatric Illnesses by Questionnaire*, London, Oxford University Press.

GOLDBERG, D. and HUXLEY, P. (1980) *Mental Illness in the Community*, London, Tavistock.

GOLDBERG, E.M. and CONNELLY, N. (1981) *Evaluative Research in Social Care*, London, Heineman.

GOLDBERG, E.M. and WHARBURTON, W. (1979) *Ends and Means in Social Work* London, George Allen and Unwin.

GOLDBERG, E., WHARBURTON, R., McGUINESS, B. and ROWLANDS, J. (1977)

'Towards accountability in social work: One year's intake to an area office', *British Journal of Social Work*, **7**, pp. 257–84.

GOULDNER, A. (1957) 'Cosmopolitans and Locals: Towards an analysis of latent social roles', *Administrative Science Quarterly*, **2**, pp. 231–300.

GREENE, J. (1968) 'The psychiatric nurse in the community', *International Journal of Nursing Studies*, **5**, pp. 175–83.

GREY, S., CORTI, P. and TATE, A. (1988) 'External Relations' in ECHLIN, R. (Ed.) *Community Mental Health Centres/Teams Information Pack*, London, Good Practices in Mental Health.

GRUBB, J. (1980) 'An Interpretation of the Johnson Behavioural System Model for Nursing Practice', in REIHL, J.P. and ROY, C. (Ed.) *Conceptual Models for Nursing Practice*, Second Edition, London, Prentice Hall.

GURIN, A. (1972) *Community Organization and Social Planning*, New York, John Wiley.

HADLEY, R. and MCGRATH, M. (1984) *When Social Services are Local: The Normanton Experience*, London, Allen and Unwin.

HAINES, J. (1981) *Skills and Methods in Social Work*, Revised Edition, London, Constable.

HAMMERSLEY, M. and ATKINSON, P. (1983) *Ethnography: Principles in Practice*, London, Tavistock.

HARDIKER, P. (1977) 'Social Work Ideologies in the Probation Service', *British Journal of Social Work*, **7**, pp. 131–54.

HARDIKER, P. (1981) 'Heart or Head. The Function and Role of Knowledge in Social Work', *Issues in Social Work Education*, **2**, 1, pp. 85–112.

HARGIE, O. and MCCARTON, P. (1986) *Social Skills Training and Psychiatric Nursing*, London, Croom Helm.

HARGREAVES, R. (1979) 'Social services for mentally ill people', in CYPHER, J. (Ed.) *Seebohm Across Three Decades*, Birmingham, BASW.

HARRE, R. (1970) *The Principles of Scientific Thinking*, London, Macmillan.

HENDERSON, A.S. (1984) 'Interpreting the evidence on social support', *Social Psychiatry*, **19**, pp. 49–52.

HENDERSON, V. (1964) *Basic Principles of Nursing Care*, Geneva, International Council of Nurses.

HENDERSON, S., BYRNE, D. and DUNCAN-JONES, P. (1981) *Neurosis in the Social Environment*, London, Academic Press.

HOGHUGHI, M. (1980) 'Social Work in a Bind', *Community Care*, 3 November, pp. 17–23.

HOLLIS, F. (1970) 'The Psychosocial Approach to the Practice of Casework', in ROBERTS, R. and NEE, R. (Eds) *Theories of Social Casework*, London, University of Chicago Press.

HOLLIS, F. (1972) *Casework: A Psychosocial Therapy*, Second Edition, New York, Random House.

HOWE, D. (1979) 'Agency Function and Social Work Principles', *British Journal of Social Work*, **9**, pp. 29–48.

HOWE, D. (1980) 'Inflated States and Empty Theories in Social Work', *British Journal of Social Work*, **10**, pp. 317–40.

HOWE, D. (1986) *Social Workers and Their Practice in Welfare Bureaucracies*, Aldershot, Gower.

HUDSON, B. (1974) 'The families of agoraphobics treated by Behaviour Therapy', *British Journal of Social Work*, **4**, 1, pp. 51–9.

HUDSON, B. (1978) 'Behavioural social work with schizophrenic patients in the community', *British Journal of Social Work*, **8**, 2, pp. 159–70.

HUDSON, B. (1982) *Social Work with Psychiatric Patients*, London, Macmillan.

HUGHES, E. (1958) *Men and Their Work*, Free Press, New York.

HUNTER, P. (1974) 'Community Psychiatric Nursing in Britain: An historical review', *International Journal of Nursing Studies*, **11**, pp. 223–33.

HUNTER, P. (1978) *Schizophrenia and Community Psychiatric Nursing*, National Schizophrenia Fellowship.

HUNTER, P. (1980) 'Social Work and Community Psychiatric Nursing — A Review', *International Journal of Nursing Studies*, **17**, pp. 131–9.

HUNTINGTON, J. (1981) *Social Work and General Medical Practice: Collaboration or Conflict*, London, George Allen and Unwin.

HUTTON, F. (1985) 'Self referrals to a Community Mental Health Centre: A three year study', *British Journal of Psychiatry*, **147**, pp. 540–4.

HUXLEY, P. and FITZPATRICK, R. (1984) 'The probable extent of minor mental illness in adult clients of social workers: a research note', *British Journal of Social Work*, **14**, pp. 67–73.

HUXLEY, P., KORER, J. and TOLLEY, S. (1987) 'The Psychiatric "Caseness" of Clients Referred to an Urban Social Services Department', *British Journal of Social Work*, **17**, pp. 507–20.

HUXLEY, P., RAVAL, H., KORER, J. and JACOB, C. (1989) 'Psychiatric morbidity in the clients of social workers: Clinical outcome', *Psychological Medicine*, **19**, pp. 189–97.

IRVING, S. (1978) *Basic Psychiatric Nursing*, London, W.B. Saunders.

ISAAC, B., MINTY, E. and MORRISON, R. (1986) 'Children in care: The association with mental disorder in the parents', *British Journal of Social Work*, **16**, pp. 325–39.

JAMOUS, H. and PELOILLE, B. (1970) 'Professions or self perpetuating systems? Changes in the French University — Hospital System' in JACKSON, J.A. (Ed.) *Professions and Socialization*, Cambridge, Cambridge Univeristy Press.

JOHNSON, D. (1980) 'The Behavioural System Model for Nursing' in REIHL, J.P. and ROY, C. (Eds) *Conceptual Models for Nursing Practice*, Second Edition, London, Prentice Hall.

JOHNSON, P. and RUBIN, A. (1983) 'Case management in mental health: A social work domain', *Social Work*, **28**, pp. 49–55.

JONES, K. (1988) *Experience in Mental Health: Community Care and Social Policy*, London, Sage.

JORDAN, W. (1979) *Helping in Social Work*, London, Routledge and Kegan Paul.

KADUSHIN, A. (1983) *The Social Work Interview*, New York, Columbia University Press.

KAGAN, C. (Ed.) (1985) *Interpersonal Skills In Nursing*, London, Croom Helm.

KAGAN, C., EVANS, J. and KAY, B. (1986) *A Manual of Interpersonal Skills for Nurses*, London, Harper and Row.

KALISCH, B. (1971) 'Strategies for developing nurses' empathy', *Nursing Outlook*, **19**, 11, pp. 714–18.

KALKMAN, M. and DAVIS, A. (Ed.) (1974) *Dimensions of Mental Health — Psychiatric Nursing*, New York, McGraw Hill.

KEAT, R. and URRY, J. (1982) *Social Theory as Science*, Second Edition, London, Routledge and Kegan Paul.

KEITH-LUCAS, A. (1972) *Giving and Taking Help*, Chapel Hill, NC, University of North Carolina Press.

KIM, H.S. (1983) *The Nature of Theoretical Thinking in Nursing*, London, Prentice Hall.

KING, I.M. (1981) *A Theory for Nursing*, London, John Wiley.

KYES, J. and HOFLING, C. (1980) *Basic Psychiatric Concepts in Nursing*, Philadelphia, J.P. Lipincott.

LANCASTER, J. (1980) *Community Mental Health Nursing: An Ecological Perspective*, London, C.V. Mosby.

LEFF, J. and VAUGHN, C. (1984) *Expressed Emotions in Families*, London, The Guildford Press.

LEONARD, P. (1975) 'Explanation and Education in Social Work', *British Journal of Social Work*, 5, pp. 325–34.

LISHMAN, J. (Ed.) (1984) *Evaluation*, Aberdeen, University of Aberdeen.

LITWACK, L., LITWACK, J. and BALLOON, M. (1980) *Health Counselling*, New York, Appleton Crofts.

LOCKER, D. and DUNT, D. (1978) 'Theoretical and Methodological Issues in Sociological Studies of Consumer Satisfaction with Medical Care', *Social Science and Medicine*, 12, pp. 283–92.

LOOMS, M. and HORSELY, J. (1974) *Interpersonal Change: A Behavioural Approach to Nursing Practice*, New York, McGraw Hill.

MARKS, I.M. (1985) *Psychiatric Nurse Therapists in Primary Care*, London, Royal College of Nursing.

MARKS, I.M., HALLAM, R.S., CONNOLLY, J. and PHILPOTT, R. (1977). *Nursing in Behavioural Psychotherapy*, London, Royal College of Nursing.

MARKS-MARAN, D. (1988) *Skills for Care Planning*, London, Skutari Press.

MARRAM, C.D. (1973) *The Group Approach to Nursing Practice*, St. Louis, C.V. Mosby.

MARSH, C. (1982) *The Survey Method: The Contribution of Surveys to Sociological Explanation*, London, Allen and Unwin.

MASLOW, A.H. (1970) *Motivation and Personality*, Second Edition, New York, Harper and Row.

McAULEY, P., CATHERWOOD, M.L., BOLTON, R. and CAMPBELL, D. (1983) 'The social work task in an acute psychiatric in-patient unit'. *British Journal of Social Work*, 13, pp. 627–38.

McFARLANE, BARONESS and CASTLEDENE, G. (1982) *A Guide to the Practice of Nursing Using the Nursing Process*, London, C.V. Mosby.

McKINLAY, J.B. (1975) *Processing People: Cases in Organizational Behaviour*, London, Holt Reinhart.

MERTON, R.K., READER, G.G. and KENDALL, P. (1957) *The Student Physician*, Cambridge, MA, Harvard University Press.

MIDDLEMAN, R. and GOLDBERG, G. (1974) *Social Service Delivery: A Structural Approach to Social Work Practice*, London, Columbia University Press.

MILES, A. (1987) *The Mentally Ill in Contemporary Society*, Second Edition, Oxford, Basil Blackwell.

MIND (1983) *Common Concern*, London, MIND.
MINISTRY OF HEALTH (1962) *A Hospital Plan for England and Wales*, London, HMSO.
MITCHELL, R. (1974) 'Medical Model versus Social Model', *Nursing Times*, **70**, 48, pp. 1851-3.
MOFFETT, J. (1968) *Concepts in Casework Treatment*, London, Routledge and Kegan Paul.
MOORE, S. (1964) 'Mental Nursing in the Community', *Nursing Times*, **60**, pp. 467-70.
MUELLER, D.P. (1980) 'Social Networks: A promising direction for research on the relationship of the social environment and psychiatric disorders', *Social Science and Medicine*, **14A**, pp. 147-61.
MUNRO, A. and McCULLOCH, J.W. (1969) *Psychiatry for Social Workers*, Oxford, Pergamon.
MUNTON, R. (1990) 'Client satisfaction with community psychiatric nursing', in BROOKER, C. (Ed.) *Community Psychiatric Nursing: A Research Perspective*, London, Routledge.
NATIONAL INSTITUTE FOR SOCIAL WORK (NISW) (1982) *Social Workers: Their Role and Tasks (Barclay Report)*, London, Bedford Square.
NEUMAN, B. (1980) 'The Betty Neuman Health-Care Systems Model', in REIHL, J.P. and ROY, C. (Ed.) *Conceptual Models for Nursing Practice*, Second Edition, London, Prentice Hall.
NEUMAN, B. (1982) *The Neuman Systems Model*, New York, Appleton Century Croft.
NURSE, G. (1975) *Counselling and the Nurse*, Aylesbury, HM and M.
OREM, D.E. (1980) *Nursing: Concepts of Practice*, Second Edition, New York, McGraw Hill.
PARNELL, J.W. (1978) *Community Psychiatric Nursing: A Descriptive Study*, London, Queens Nursing Institute.
PATERSON, J.G. and ZDERAD, L.T. (1976) *Humanistic Nursing*, New York, John Wiley and Son.
PAVALKO, R. (1971) *The Sociology of Occupations*, Itasca, IL, Peacock.
PAYKEL, E.S. and GRIFFITHS, J.H. (1983) *Community Psychiatric Nursing for Neurotic Patients*, London, Royal College of Nursing.
PEARSON, A. and VAUGHN, B. (1984) *Nursing Models for Practice*, London, Heinemann.
PECK, E. and JOYCE, L. (1985) 'Community Mental Health Centres — A View of the Landscape' in McAUSLAND, T. (Ed.) *Planning and Monitoring Community Mental Health Centres*, Kings Fund, Unpublished.
PEPLEAU, H.E. (1962) 'Interpersonal techniques: The crux of psychiatric nursing', *American Journal of Nursing*, **62**, pp. 50-4.
PEPLEAU, H.E. (1980) The Psychiatric Nurse — Accountable? to whom? for what? *Perspectives in Psychiatric Care*, **18**, pp. 128-34.
PEPLEAU, H. (1988) *Interpersonal Relations in Nursing*, Second Edition, London, Macmillan.
PERLMAN, H.H. (1957) *Social Casework: A Problem Solving Process*, Chicago, University of Chicago Press.
PERLMAN, H.H. (1969) 'Foreword' to REID, W. and SHYNE, A., *Brief and Extended Casework*, London, Columbia University Press.

PERLMAN, H. (1970) 'The Problem Solving Model in Social Casework', in ROBERTS, R. and NEE, R. (Eds) *Theories of Social Casework*, London, University of Chicago Press.

PERLMAN, H. (1979) *Relationship: The Heart of Helping People*, Chicago, University of Chicago Press.

PHILLIPS, D. (1983) 'Mayer and Timms revisited: The evaluation of client studies', in FISHER, M. (Ed.) *Speaking of Clients*, Sheffield, JUSSR, University of Sheffield Press.

PINCUS, A. and MINAHAN, A. (1975) *Social Work Practice: Model and Method*, Itasca, IL, Peacock.

PIPPIN, J. (1980) *Developing Casework Skills*, London, Sage.

POPE, B. (1986) *Social Skills Training for Psychiatric Nurses*, London, Harper and Row.

PORRITT, L. (1984) *Communication: Choices for Nurses*, London, Churchill Livingstone.

POWELL, J. ENOCH (1961) *Report of the Annual Conference of the National Association for Mental Health*, London.

PUTTNAM, M. (1981) 'Medical and Social Models'. *Nursing Times*, **77**, 19, pp. 832.

RAGG, N. (1977) *People Not Cases*, London, Routledge and Kegan Paul.

RAMBO, B.J. (1984) *Adaptation Nursing*, London, W.B. Saunders.

RAPPAPORT, L. (1970) 'Crisis Intervention as a Mode of Brief Treatment' in ROBERTS, R.W. and NEE, R.H. (Eds) *Theories of Social Casework*, Chicago, Chicago University Press.

REED, V. (1988) 'Community Nursing in Mental Disorder' in MALIN, N. (Ed.) *Reassessing Community Care*, London, Croom Helm.

REES, S. (1974) 'No more than contact: An outcome of social work', British Journal of Social Work, **4**, pp. 255–79.

REES, S. (1978) *Social Work Face to Face*, London, Edward Arnold.

REES, S. and WALLACE, A. (1982) *Verdicts in Social Work*, London, Edward Arnold.

REID, W. (1978) *The Task Centred System*, New York, Columbia University Press.

REID, W.J. and EPSTEIN, L. (1972) *Task Control Casework*, London, Columbia University Press.

REID, W.J. and SHYNE, A. (1969) *Brief and Extended Casework*, London, Columbia University Press.

REIHL, J.P. and ROY, C. (Eds) (1980) *Conceptual Models for Nursing*, Second Edition, London, Prentice Hall.

REYNOLDS, B. (1985) 'Issues arising from teaching interpersonal skills in psychiatric nurse training', in KEGAN, C. (Ed.) *Interpersonal Skills in Nursing*, London, Croom Helm.

RITTER, S. (1989) *Bethlem Royal and Mandsley Hospital Manual of Clinical Psychiatric Nursing — Principles and Procedures*, London, Harper and Row.

ROACH, F. and FARLEY, N. (1986) 'The Behavioural Management of Neurosis by the Psychiatric Nurse Therapist', in BROOKING, J. (Ed.) *Psychiatric Nursing Research*, Chichester, John Wiley.

ROBERTS, R. and NEE, R. (1970) *Theories of Social Casework*, London, University of Chicago Press.

ROGERS, M.E. (1970) *An Introduction to the Theoretical Basis of Nursing*, Philadelphia, F.A. Davis.

ROPER, N., LOGAN, W. and TIERNEY, A. (1980) *The Elements of Nursing*, London, Churchill Livingstone.

ROPER, N., LOGAN, W. and TIERNEY, A.J. (1981) *Learning to Use the Process of Nursing*, Edinburgh, Churchill Livingstone.

ROY, C. (1975) 'A diagnostic classification system for nursing', *Nursing Outlook*, **23**, pp. 90–4.

ROY, C. (1976) *Introduction to Nursing: An Adaptation Model*, Englewood Cliffs, NJ, Prentice Hall.

ROY, C. and ROBERTS, S.L. (1981) *Theory Construction in Nursing: An Adaptation Model*, Englewood Cliffs, NJ, Prentice Hall.

RUBINGTON, E. and WEINBERG, M. (1977) *The Study of Social Problems*, New York, Oxford University Press.

RUSHFORTH, D. (1990) 'Recruitment to post basic CPN certificate courses in the United Kingdom for 1989–90', *Community Psychiatric Nursing Journal*, **10**, 2, pp. 17–20.

RUSHTON, A. and BRISCOE, M. (1981) 'Social Work as an Aspect of Primary Health Care: The Social Workers' View', *British Journal of Social Work*, **11**, pp. 61–76.

SAINSBURY, E. (1970) *Social Diagnosis in Casework*, London, Routledge and Kegan Paul.

SAINSBURY, E. (1975) *Social Work with Families*, London, Routledge and Kegan Paul.

SAINSBURY, E. (1977) *The Personal Social Services*, London, Pitman.

SAINSBURY, E., NIXON, S. and PHILLIPS, D. (1982) *Social Work in Focus*, London, Routledge and Kegan Paul.

SATIR, V. (1964) *Conjoint Family Therapy: A Guide to Therapy and Technique*, Palo Alto, CA, Science and Behaviour Books.

SAYCE, L. (1987) 'Revolution under Review', *The Health Service Journal*, **97**, 5078, pp. 1378–9.

SAYCE, L. (Ed.) (1988) *Community Mental Health Centres: Report of the Annual Conference 1987*, Unpublished. NUPRD.

SAYCE, L. (1989) 'Community Mental Health Centres — Rhetoric and Reality' in BRACKX, A. and GRIMSHAW, C. (Eds) *Mental Health Care in Crisis*, London, Pluto Press.

SEEBOHM, F. (1968) *Report of the Committee on Local Authority and Allied Personal Social Services*, London, HMSO.

SHELDON, B. (1978) 'Theory and Practice in Social Work — A Re-examination of a Tenuous Relationship', *British Journal of Social Work*, **8**, 1, pp. 1–22.

SHELDON, B. (1982) *Behavioural Modification*, London, Tavistock.

SHELDON, B. (1983) 'The Use of Single Case Experimental Designs in the Evaluation of Social Work', *British Journal of Social Work*, No. 13, pp. 477–500.

SHEPHERD, M., HARWIN, B.G., DEPLA, C. and CAIRNS, V. (1979) 'Social work and the primary care of mental disorder', *Psychological Medicine*, **9**, pp. 661–9.

SHEPPARD, M. (1982) *Perceptions of Child Abuse: A Critique of Individualism*, Norwich, UEA Press.

SHEPPARD, M. (1984) 'Notes on the use of social explanation to social work', *Issues in Social Work Education*, **4**, pp. 27–42.

SHEPPARD, M. (1987) 'Dominant Images of Social Work: A British comparison of general practitioners with and without attachment schemes', *International Social Work*, **30**, 1, pp. 77–91.

SHEPPARD, M. (1990) *Mental Health: The Role of the Approved Social Worker*, Sheffield, JUSSR, University of Sheffield Press.

SHORT, R. (1985) *Second Report of the Social Services Committee: Community Care*, Vol. I to III, London, HMSO.

SHULMAN, L. (1984) *The Skills of Helping*, Itasca, IL, F.E. Peacock.

SIBEON, R. (1982) 'Theory-practice symbolization: A critical review of the Hardiker-Davies debate', *Issues in Social Work Education*, **2**, pp. 119–47.

SIEGLER, M. and OSMOND, H. (1966) 'Models of Madness', *British Journal of Psychiatry*, **112**, pp. 1193–203.

SILVERMAN, D. (1985) *Qualitative Methodology and Sociology: Describing the Social World*, Aldershot, Gower.

SIMMONS, S. and BROOKER, C. (1986) *Community Psychiatric Nursing: A Social Perspective*, London, Heinemann.

SIMPSON, I. (1967) 'Patterns of socialization into professions: The case of student nurses', *Sociological Inquiry*, **37**, pp. 47–54.

SIPORIN, M. (1975) *Introduction to Social Work Practice*, New York, Macmillan.

SKIDMORE, D. (1985) 'More chalk than talk', *Community Outlook*, September, 12–13.

SKIDMORE, D. and FRIEND, W. (1984) 'Muddling through', *Community Outlook*, 9 May, pp. 179–81.

SLADDEN, S. (1979) *Psychiatric Nursing in the Community*, London, Churchill Livingstone.

SMALE, G., TUSON, G., COOPER, M., WARDLE, M. and CROSBIE, D. (1988) *Community Social Work: A Paradigm for Change*, London, National Institute of Social Work.

SMITH, G. and HARRIS, R. (1972) 'Ideologies of Need and the Organization of Social Work Departments', *British Journal of Social Work*, **2**, pp. 27–45.

SMITH, H.W. (1975) *Strategies of Social Research*, Englewood Cliffs, NJ, Prentice Hall.

SMITH, V. and BASS, T. (1982) *Communication for the Health Care Team*, London, Harper and Row.

SPECHT H. and VICKERY, A. (1978) *Integrating Social Work Methods*, London, George Allen and Unwin.

SPEIGHT, T. (1986) 'Communicating with Psychiatric Patients', in BRIDGE, W. and MCLEOD-CLARK, J. (Eds) *Communication in Nursing Care*

STACEY, M. (1969) *Methods of Social Research*, London, Pergamon Press.

STEVENS, B. (1979) *Nursing Theory: Analysis, Application, Evaluation*, Boston, Little Brown.

STEVENSON, O. (1971) 'Knowledge for Social Work', *British Journal of Social Work*, 1, **2**, pp. 225–7.

STEWART, W. (1975) 'Nursing and Counselling — A Conflict of Roles', *Nursing Mirror*, **14**, p. 171.

STEWART, W. (1983) *Counselling in Nursing: A Problem Solving Approach*, London, Harper and Row.

STEWART, W. (1985) *Counselling in Rehabilitation*, Beckenham, Croom Helm.

STRAUSS, A., SCHATZMAN, L., EHRLICH, D., BUCHER, R. and SABSHIN, M. (1964) *Psychiatric Ideologies and Institutions*, New York, Free Press.

STUART, G.W. and SUNDEEN, S.J. (1983) *Principles and Practice of Psychiatric Nursing*, London, C.V. Mosby.

TIMMS, N. (1964) *Social Casework*, London, Routledge and Kegan Paul.

THYER, B.A. (1987) *Treating Anxiety Disorders*, London, Sage.

TRICK, K. and OBCORSKAS, A. (1980) *Understanding Mental Illness and its Nursing*, Tunbridge Wells, Pitman.

TRUAX, C. and CARKHUFF, R. (1967) *Towards Effective Counselling and Psychotherapy*, Chicago, Aldine.

TSCHUDIN, V. (1987) *Counselling Skills for Nurses*, London, Balliere-Tindall.

TYRER, P. and STEINBERG, P. (1987) *Models for Mental Disorder*, Chichester, John Wiley.

WIS (1989) *Internal Document*, Unpublished.

WALTON, H. (1984) 'Medicine', in GOODLAD, S. (Ed.) *Education for the Professions*, Guildford, NFER-Nelson.

WARD, M. (1985) *The Nursing Process in Psychiatry*, London, Churchill Livingstone.

WARD, M. and BISHOP, R. (1988) *Learning to Care in Community Psychiatric Nursing*, Bungay, Chaucer Press.

WEBER, R.P. (1985) *Basic Content Analysis*, London, Sage.

WEISS, C. (1972) *Evaluation Research*, Englewood Cliffs, NJ, Prentice Hall.

WHITTAKER, J.K. (1974) *Social Treatment*, Chicago, Aldine.

WHITTAKER, J.K. (1986) 'Integrating formal and informal care: a conceptual framework', *British Journal of Social Work*, Supplement, pp. 39–62.

WHITTAKER, J.K. and GABARINO, J. (1983) *Social Support Networks*, New York, Aldine.

WING, J.K., COOPER, J.E. and SARTORIOUS, N. (1974) *The Measurement and Classification of Psychiatric Symptoms: An Introduction Manual of the Present State Examination and CATEGO Programme*, London, Cambridge University Press.

WOOFF, K. (1987) *A Comparison of the Work of Community Psychiatric Nurses and Mental Health Social Worker in Salford*, PhD, University of Manchester.

WOOFF, K. and GOLDBERG, D. (1988) 'Further observations on the practice of community care in Salford', *British Journal of Psychiatry*, 153, pp. 30–7.

WOOFF, K., GOLDBERG, D.P. and FRYERS, T. (1986) 'Patients in receipt of community psychiatric nursing care in Salford, 1976–82', *Psychological Medicine*, 16, pp. 407–14.

WOOFF, K., GOLDBERG, D.P. and FRYERS, T. (1988a) 'The Practice of Community Psychiatric Nursing and Mental Health Social Work in Salford: Some Implications for Community Care', *British Journal of Psychiatry*, 152, pp. 783–92.

WOOFF, K. and GOLDBERG, D.P. (1988b) 'Further observations on the practice of community care in Salford: Difference between community psychiatric nurses and mental health social workers', *British Journal of Psychiatry*, 153, pp. 30–7.

WOOTTON, B. (1959) *Social Science and Social Pathology*, London, George Allen and Unwin.

WORLD HEALTH ORGANIZATION (WHO) (1977) *Manual of the International Statistical Classification of Diseases, Injuries and Causes of Death*, Volumes, London, HMSO.

YELLOLY, M. (1980) *Social Work Theory and Psychoanalysis*, London, Van Nostrand Reinehold.

YUEN, R. (1984) 'The nurse–client relationship: a mutual learning experience', *Journal of Advanced Nursing*, **11**, pp. 529–35.

Index